Color Atlas
of Oral Diseases

Color Atlas of Oral Diseases

George Laskaris, D.D.S., M.D.

Foreword by Gerald Shklar
491 Illustrations

1988
Georg Thieme Verlag
Stuttgart · New York

Thieme Medical Publishers, Inc.
New York

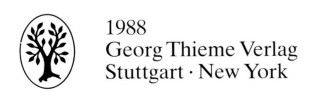
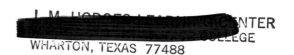

George Laskaris, D.D.S., M.D.
Associate Professor in Oral Medicine and Pathology,
Dental School, University of Athens.
Consultant in Oral Medicine,
Dept. of Dermatology, «A. Syngros» Hospital,
University of Athens.
20–22 Ipsilandou St.
10676 Athens, Greece

Library of Congress Cataloging-in-Publication-Data

Laskaris. George.
  [Enchromos atlas stomatologias. English]
  Color atlas of oral diseases / George Laskaris :
  foreword by
Gerald Shklar.
    p. cm.
  Translation of: Enchromos atlas stomatologias.
  Bibliography: p.
  Includes index.
  ISBN 0-86577-297-5 (Thieme Medical Publishers)
  1. Mouth--Diseases--Atlases. I. Title.
  [DNLM: 1. Mouth Diseases--atlases. WU 17 L345e]
RC815.L3713 1988
617'.522--dc19
DNLM/DLC
for Library of Congress   88-16090
                                                      CIP

Important Note: Medicine is an ever-changing science. Research and clinical experience are continually broadening our knowledge, in particular our knowledge of proper treatment and drug therapy. Insofar as this book mentions any dosage or application, readers may rest assured that the authors, editors and publishers have made every effort to ensure that such references are strictly in accordance with the state of knowledge at the time of production of the book. Nevertheless, every user is requested to carefully examine the manufacturers' leaflets accompanying each drug to check on his own responsibility whether the dosage schedules recommended therein or the contraindications stated by the manufacturers differ from the statements made in the present book. Such examination is particularly important with drugs which are either rarely used or have been newly released on the market.

This atlas is based on the Greek edition:
Enchromos Atlas Stomatologias –
Color Atlas of Stomatology
Copyright © 1986 by George Laskaris, Athens, Greece.
Published by Litsas Medical Publications,
Athens, Greece

Cover design: Renate Stockinger

© 1988 Georg Thieme Verlag, Rüdigerstraße 14, D-7000 Stuttgart 30, West Germany
Thieme Medical Publishers, Inc.,
381 Park Avenue South, New York, N. Y. 10016

Typesetting by Druckhaus Dörr, D-7140 Ludwigsburg (System 5, Linotron 202)
Printed in West Germany by Druckerei Appl,
D-8853 Wemding

ISBN 3-13-717001-X (Georg Thieme Verlag, Stuttgart)
ISBN 0-86577-297-5 (Thieme Medical Publishers, Inc., New York)

                                          1 2 3 4 5 6

Foreword

It is a distinct pleasure to see Dr. George Laskaris' excellent Atlas of Oral Diseases come out in an English edition. Dr. Laskaris' knowledge, background, and wealth of experience in the disciplines of oral medicine and oral pathology have been well known to those of us in the field. His highly respected research on autoimmune diseases of the mouth has appeared in many English language journals, and it is fitting that his extensive experience with oral diseases is now made available to the English-speaking world. This Atlas has impressed even those of us who could not read the original Greek, by the excellence of the color illustrations and the broad range of diseases covered. The English text now offers a brief but authoritative discussion of each condition.

GERALD SHKLAR, D.D.S, M.S.
Charles A. Brackett Professor of Oral Pathology
and Head of the Department of Oral Medicine
and Oral Pathology,
Harvard School of Dental Medicine,
Boston, Massachusetts

Preface

Oral medicine is a rapidly growing clinical specialty encompassing the diagnosis and treatment of patients with a wide spectrum of disorders involving the oral cavity.

To achieve the optimum goals, oral medical clinicians have to broaden their knowledge bases and practise their clinical skills.

When I first started to work in this field 20 years ago, I could not imagine the variety of disorders that affect the oral cavity, including genetic diseases, infections, cancers, blood diseases, skin diseases, endocrine and metabolic disorders, autoimmune and rheumatologic diseases, local lesions, to name a few. Fortunately, the oral cavity is accessible to visual examination, and I have attempted to record oral lesions in color slides. During my career as a stomatologist, I have collected more than 25,000 clinical color slides that encompass a broad spectrum of common and rare oral diseases. The most representative and educationally useful illustrations have been used in this Atlas. Almost all color slides have been taken by me with a Nikon-Medical camera.

This book is the distillation of my clinical experience and is intended to aid primarily the practicing dentist, the specialist in oral medicine, the oral pathologist and surgeon, the dermatologist, and otorhinolaryngologist to solve the diagnostic problems posed by oral diseases. It can also be valuable to dental and medical students, general internists, pediatricians, and other medical specialists.

This book is not a complete reference work of oral medicine and should be used in conjunction with current textbooks and articles regarding recommendations on treatment and new diagnostic techniques that are beyond its scope.

The material of the Atlas is divided into 33 chapters. Each entity is accompanied by color plates and a description of the clinical features, differential diagnosis, helpful laboratory tests, and a brief statement on treatment.

Selective bibliography and index are included.

I hope that the Atlas will serve as a comprehensive pictorial guide for diagnostic problems in the mouth and it will find its way in the places where the battle against oral diseases is waged daily, that is dental schools, hospitals, and private practice offices.

Athens, 1988   GEORGE LASKARIS

Acknowledgments

My deep appreciation is due to my patients, who taught me so much, and to all Greek dentists and physicians who have contributed by referring their patients to me through the years.

My gratitude is extended to the late Professor of Dermatology John Kapetanakis and the current Professor of Dermatology and Head of the Department of Dermatology, University of Athens, "A. Syngros" Hospital, John Stratigos, for their constant encouragement in my endeavors.

I am also indebted to Associate Professor of Dermatology Antony Vareltzidis who has greatly helped me to broaden my knowledge in the field of Dermatology.

My sincere thanks are extended to the scientific staff of "A. Syngros" Hospital, Department of Dermatology, University of Athens, for their willing and prompt help during the 18 years of our cooperation.

I am particularly grateful to Stathis S. Papavasiliou, M.D., for his efforts and comments on the translation of the Greek edition of this book into English and text contributions in the chapter of endocrine diseases.

My deepest gratitude is due to Professor Crispian Scully, Department of Oral Medicine and Surgery, University of Bristol, England and Professor Gerald Shklar, Department of Oral Medicine and Pathology, Harvard School of Dental Medicine, United States, both of whom read the manuscript. Their suggestions and criticisms have been gratefully received and indeed improved the text considerably.

Finally, I wish to thank my colleagues at the Department of Oral Medicine and Pathology of the Dental School, University of Athens, with whom I have worked closely for more than 20 years. In particular I wish to thank Dr. Alexandra Sklavounou, Dr. Panagiota Economopoulou, and Dr. Eleana Stufi for their assistance in the preparation of the Atlas.

I thank the following colleagues for permission to use their color plates: Dr. Robert Gorlin (USA) for Figure 43, Dr. Nikos Lygidakis (Greece) for Figure 61, Dr. Adeyeni Mosadomi (Nigeria) for Figure 424, Dr. Gerald Shklar (USA) for Figures 231, 232, 339, and Dr. Carl Witkop (USA) for Figure 20.

Last, but by no means least, I can never fully repay all that I owe my wife and three children for their constant patience, support, and encouragement.

Contents

1. Normal Anatomic Variants 2

Linea Alba 2
Normal Oral Pigmentation 2
Leukoedema 2

2. Developmental Anomalies 4

Fordyce's Granules 4
Congenital Lip Pits 4
Ankyloglossia 4
Cleft Lip 6
Cleft Palate 6
Bifid Tongue 6
Double Lip 8
Torus Palatinus 8
Torus Mandibularis 8
Multiple Exostoses 8
Fibrous Developmental Malformation 10
Facial Hemiatrophy 10
Masseteric Hypertrophy 10

3. Genetic Diseases 12

White Sponge Nevus 12
Hereditary Benign Intraepithelial
Dyskeratosis 12
Gingival Fibromatosis 12
Pachyonychia Congenita 14
Dyskeratosis Congenita 14
Hypohidrotic Ectodermal Dysplasia 16
Focal Palmoplantar and Oral Mucosa
Hyperkeratosis Syndrome 16
Papillon-Lefèvre Syndrome 18
Benign Acanthosis Nigricans 18
Dyskeratosis Follicularis 20
Familial Benign Pemphigus 20
Epidermolysis Bullosa 22
Neurofibromatosis 24
Chondroectodermal Dysplasia 24
Hereditary Hemorrhagic Telangiectasia . . . 26
Peutz-Jeghers Syndrome 26
Maffucci's Syndrome 26

Tuberous Sclerosis 28
Sturge-Weber Syndrome 28
Klippel-Trenaunay-Weber Syndrome 30
Cowden's Disease 30
Cleidocranial Dysplasia 32
Oro-Facial Digital Syndrome 32
Focal Dermal Hypoplasia 34
Incontinentia Pigmenti 34
Ehlers-Danlos Syndrome 36

4. Mechanical Injuries 38

Traumatic Ulcer 38
Traumatic Hematoma 40
Chronic Biting 40
Toothbrush Trauma 40
Factitious Trauma 40
Fellatio 42
Lingual Frenum Ulcer After Cunnilingus . . 42
Cotton Roll Stomatitis 42
Denture Stomatitis 44
Epulis Fissuratum 44
Papillary Hyperplasia of the Palate 44
Hyperplasia due to Negative Pressure 46
Atrophy of the Maxillary Alveolar Ridge . . 46
Foreign Body Reaction 46
Palatal Necrosis due to Injection 48
Eosinophilic Ulcer 48

5. Oral Lesions due to Chemical Agents . . . 50

Phenol Burn 50
Trichloroacetic Acid Burn 50
Eugenol Burn 50
Aspirin Burn 52
Iodine Burn 52
Alcohol Burn 52
Acrylic Resin Burn 52
Sodium Perborate Burn 54
Silver Nitrate Burn 54
Sodium Hypochlorite Burn 54
Paraformaldehyde Burn 54

6. Oral Lesions due to Heat 56

Nicotinic Stomatitis 56
Palatal Erosions due to Smoking 56
Cigarette Smoker's Lip Lesion 58
Thermal Burn 58

7. Oral Lesions due to Drugs 60

Gold-Induced Stomatitis 60
Antibiotic-Induced Stomatitis 60
Stomatitis Medicamentosa 60
Ulcerations due to Methotrexate 62
Ulceration due to Azathioprine 62
Penicillamine-Induced Oral Lesions 62
Fibrous Gingival Hyperplasia due to
Phenytoin 64
Fibrous Gingival Hyperplasia due to
Cyclosporine 64
Angioneurotic Edema 64
Pigmentation due to Antimalarials 66
Cheilitis due to Retinoids 66

8. Metal and Other Deposits 68

Amalgam Tattoo 68
Bismuth Deposition 68
Materia Alba of the Attached Gingiva 68

9. Radiation-Induced Injuries 70

**10. Allergy to Chemical Agents Applied
Locally** 72

Allergic Stomatitis due to Acrylic Resin . . . 72
Allergic Stomatitis due to Eugenol 72

11. Periodontal Diseases 74

Gingivitis 74
Periodontitis 74
Juvenile Periodontitis 74
Periodontal Abscess 76
Periodontal Fistula 76
Gingivitis and Mouth Breathing 76
Plasma Cell Gingivitis 78
Desquamative Gingivitis 78

12. Diseases of the Tongue 80

Median Rhomboid Glossitis 80
Geographic Tongue 80
Fissured Tongue 82
Hairy Tongue 82
Plasma Cell Glossitis 84

Glossodynia 84
Crenated Tongue 84
Hypertrophy of Foliate Papillae 86
Hypertrophy of Circumvallate Papillae 86
Hypertrophy of the Fungiform Papillae 86
Sublingual Varices 86

13. Diseases of the Lips 88

Angular Cheilitis 88
Actinic Cheilitis 88
Exfoliative Cheilitis 88
Contact Cheilitis 90
Cheilitis Glandularis 90
Cheilitis Granulomatosa 90
Plasma Cell Cheilitis 92

14. Soft Tissue Cysts 93

Mucocele 93
Ranula 94
Lymphoepithelial Cyst 94
Dermoid Cyst 96
Eruption Cyst 96
Gingival Cyst of the Newborn 96
Gingival Cyst of the Adult 98
Palatine Papilla Cyst 98
Thyroglossal Duct Cyst 98

15. Viral Infections 100

Primary Herpetic Gingivostomatitis 100
Secondary Herpetic Stomatitis 100
Herpes Labialis 102
Herpes Zoster 102
Varicella 104
Herpangina 104
Acute Lymphonodular Pharyngitis 104
Hand-Foot-and-Mouth Disease 106
Measles 106
Infectious Mononucleosis 108
Verruca Vulgaris 108
Condyloma Acuminatum 108
Molluscum Contagiosum 110
Focal Epithelial Hyperplasia 110
Acquired Immune Deficiency Syndrome . . . 112

16. Bacterial Infections 117

Acute Necrotizing Ulcerative Gingivitis . . . 117
Acute Necrotizing Ulcerative Stomatitis . . . 118
Cancrum Oris 118
Streptococcal Gingivostomatitis 118
Erysipelas 120
Scarlet Fever 120

Oral Soft Tissue Abscess 120
Acute Suppurative Parotitis 122
Acute Submandibular Sialadenitis 122
Buccal Cellulitis 122
Syphilis 124
    Primary Syphilis 124
    Secondary Syphilis 124
    Late Syphilis 128
Congenital Syphilis 130
Chancroid 130
Gonococcal Stomatitis 130
Tuberculosis 132
Lupus Vulgaris 134
Leprosy 134
Actinomycosis 136

17. Fungal Infections 138

Candidosis 138
    Acute Pseudomembranous Candidosis
    (Thrush) 138
    Acute Atrophic Candidosis 138
    Chronic Atrophic Candidosis 138
    Chronic Hyperplastic Candidosis, or
    Candidal Leukoplakia 138
    Chronic Multifocal Candidosis 140
    Papillary Hyperplasia of the Palate 140
    Chronic Mucocutaneous Candidosis 142
    Candida-Endocrinopathy Syndrome 142
Histoplasmosis 144
North American Blastomycosis 144

18. Other Infections 146

Cutaneous Leishmaniasis 146
Sarcoidosis 146
Heerfordt's Syndrome 148

19. Diseases with Possible
    Immunopathogenesis 149

Recurrent Aphthous Ulcers 149
    Minor Aphthous Ulcers 149
    Major Aphthous Ulcers 150
    Herpetiform Ulcers 150
Behçet's Syndrome 152
Reiter's Syndrome 154
Wegener's Granulomatosis 156
Lethal Midline Granuloma 156
Crohn's Disease 158

20. Autoimmune Diseases 159

Discoid Lupus Erythematosus 159
Systemic Lupus Erythematosus 160

Scleroderma 160
Dermatomyositis 162
Sjögren's Syndrome 164
Benign Lymphoepithelial Lesion 164
Primary Biliary Cirrhosis 164
Lupoid Hepatitis 166

21. Skin Diseases 167

Erythema Multiforme 167
Stevens-Johnson Syndrome 168
Toxic Epidermal Necrolysis 170
Pemphigus 172
    Pemphigus Vulgaris 172
    Pemphigus Vegetans 174
    Pemphigus Foliaceus 174
    Pemphigus Erythematosus 174
Juvenile Pemphigus Vulgaris 176
Cicatricial Pemphigoid 176
Cicatricial Pemphigoid of Childhood 178
Linear Immunoglobulin A Disease 180
Bullous Pemphigoid 180
Dermatitis Herpetiformis 182
Epidermolysis Bullosa Acquisita 182
Lichen Planus 184
Psoriasis 188
Mucocutaneous Lymph Node Syndrome . . . 188
Malignant Acanthosis Nigricans 190
Acrodermatitis Enteropathica 190
Perioral Dermatitis 192
Warty Dyskeratoma 192
Vitiligo 192

22. Hematologic Disorders 194

Iron Deficiency Anemia 194
Plummer-Vinson Syndrome 194
Pernicious Anemia 194
Thalassemias 196
Cyclic Neutropenia 196
Agranulocytosis 196
Aplastic Anemia 198
Thrombocytopenic Purpura 198

23. Metabolic Diseases 200

Amyloidosis 200
Lipoid Proteinosis 202
Xanthomas 202
Porphyrias 204
Hemochromatosis 204
Cystic Fibrosis 206
Histiocytosis X 206

24. Nutritional Disorders 209

Pellagra 209
Ariboflavinosis 209
Scurvy 210
Protein Deficiency 210

25. Endocrine Diseases 212

Diabetes Mellitus 212
Adrenocortical Insufficiency 212
Hypothyroidism 212
Primary Hyperparathyroidism 214
Sex Hormone Disorders 214

**26. Diseases of the Peripheral Nervous
System** 216

Hypoglossal Nerve Paralysis 216
Peripheral Facial Nerve Paralysis 216
Melkersson-Rosenthal Syndrome 218

27. Precancerous Lesions 219

Leukoplakia 219
Erythroplasia 224
Candidal Leukoplakia 224

28. Precancerous Conditions 226

Plummer-Vinson Syndrome 226
Atrophic Glossitis in Tertiary Syphilis 226
Submucous Fibrosis 226
Xeroderma Pigmentosum 228
Lichen Planus 228

29. Malignant Neoplasms 230

Squamous Cell Carcinoma 230
Verrucous Carcinoma 234
Adenoid Squamous Cell Carcinoma 236
Spindle Cell Carcinoma 236
Lymphoepithelial Carcinoma 236
Basal Cell Carcinoma 238
Acinic Cell Tumor 238
Mucoepidermoid Tumor 240
Adenoid Cystic Carcinoma 240
Malignant Pleomorphic Adenoma 240
Adenocarcinoma 242
Clear Cell Adenocarcinoma 242
Lobular Carcinoma of Minor Salivary
Glands 242
Fibrosarcoma 244
Kaposi's Sarcoma 244
Malignant Fibrous Histiocytoma 246

Hemangioendothelioma 246
Hemangiopericytoma 246
Malignant Melanoma 248
Chondrosarcoma 248
Osteosarcoma 248
Metastatic Tumors 250

**30. Malignancies of the Hematopoietic and
Lymphatic Tissues** 252

Leukemias 252
    Acute Leukemias 252
    Chronic Leukemias 254
Erythroleukemia 256
Polycythemia Vera 256
Hodgkin's Disease 256
Non-Hodgkin's Lymphomas 258
Burkitt's Lymphoma 258
Mycosis Fungoides 260
Macroglobulinemia 260
Plasmacytoma of the Oral Mucosa 262
Multiple Myeloma 262

31. Benign Tumors 264

Papilloma 264
Verrucous Hyperplasia 264
Keratoacanthoma 266
Fibroma 266
Giant Cell Fibroma 268
Peripheral Ossifying Fibroma 268
Lipoma 268
Myxoma 270
Neurofibroma 270
Schwannoma 270
Traumatic Neuroma 272
Leiomyoma 272
Verruciform Xanthoma 272
Granular Cell Tumor 274
Benign Fibrous Histiocytoma 274
Hemangioma 274
Lymphangioma 276
Cystic Hygroma 278
Papillary Syringadenoma of the Lower Lip . . 278
Sebaceous Adenoma 278
Cutaneous Horn 280
Freckles 280
Lentigo Simplex 280
Intramucosal Nevus 282
Junctional Nevus 282
Compound Nevus 282
Blue Nevus 284
Nevus of Ota 284
Lentigo Maligna 286

Melanotic Neuroectodermal Tumor of
Infancy 286
Pleomorphic Adenoma 288
Papillary Cystadenoma Lymphomatosum . . 288

32. Other Salivary Glands Disorders 290

Necrotizing Sialometaplasia 290
Sialolithiasis 290
Mikulicz's Syndrome 290
Xerostomia 292

33. Tumorlike Lesions 293

Pyogenic Granuloma 293
Pregnancy Granuloma 293
Postextraction Granuloma 294
Fistula Granuloma 294
Peripheral Giant Cell Granuloma 296
Congenital Epulis of the Newborn 296

Selected Bibliography 299

Index 315

This atlas is dedicated
to the memory of my father
and
to my family

1. Normal Anatomic Variants

Linea Alba

Linea alba is a normal linear elevation of the buccal mucosa extending from the corner of the mouth to the third molars at the occlusal line. Clinically, it presents as a bilateral linear elevation with normal or slightly whitish color and normal consistency on palpation (Fig. **1**).

It occurs more often in obese persons. The oral mucosa is slightly compressed and adjusts to the shape of the occlusal line of the teeth.

Normal Oral Pigmentation

Melanin is a normal skin and oral mucosa pigment produced by melanocytes. Increased melanin deposition in the oral mucosa may occur in various diseases. However, areas of dark discoloration may often be a normal finding in black or dark-skinned persons. However, the degree of pigmentation of skin and oral mucosa are not necessarily significant. In healthy persons there may be clinically asymptomatic black or brown areas of varying size and distribution in the oral cavity, usually on the gingiva, buccal mucosa, palate, and less often on the tongue, floor of the mouth, and lips (Fig. **2**). The pigmentation is more prominent in areas of pressure or friction and becomes more intense with aging.

The differential diagnosis includes Addison's disease, pigmented nevus, melanoma, heavy metal deposition, lentigo maligna, and pigmentation caused by drugs.

Leukoedema

Leukoedema is a normal anatomic variant of the oral mucosa due to increased thickness of the epithelium and intracellular edema of the malpighian layer. As a rule, it occurs bilaterally and involves most of the buccal mucosa and rarely the lips and tongue. Clinically, the mucosa has an opalescent or grayish-white color with slight wrinkling, which disappears if the mucosa is distended by pulling or stretching of the cheek (Fig. **3**). Leukoedema has normal consistency on palpation, and it should not be confused with leukoplakia or lichen planus.

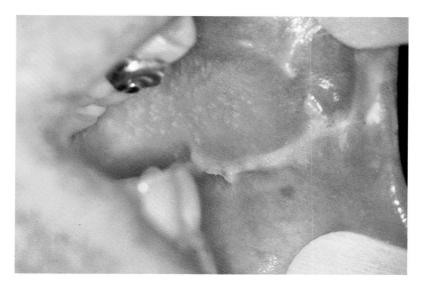

Fig. **1**. Linea alba.

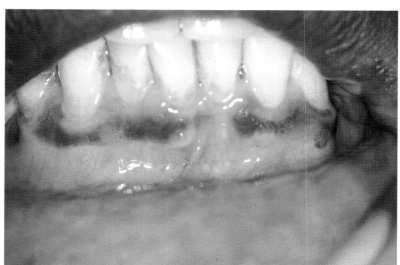

Fig. **2**. Normal pigmentation of the gingiva.

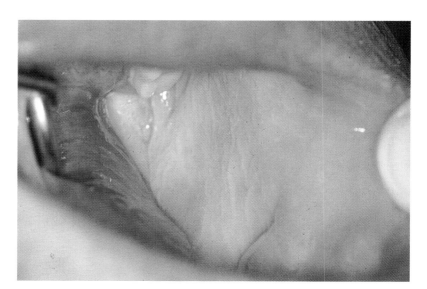

Fig. **3**. Leukoedema of the buccal mucosa.

2. Developmental Anomalies

Fordyce's Granules

Fordyce's granules are a developmental anomaly characterized by collections of heterotopic sebaceous glands in the oral mucosa. Clinically, there are many small, slightly raised whitish-yellow spots that are well circumscribed and rarely coalesce, forming plaques (Fig. 4). They occur most often in the mucosal surface of the upper lip, commissures, and the buccal mucosa adjacent to the molar teeth in a symmetrical bilateral pattern.

They are a frequent finding in about 80% of persons of both sexes. These granules are asymptomatic and come to the patient's attention by chance. With advancing age, they may become more prominent but should not be a cause for concern.

The differential diagnosis includes lichen planus, candidosis, and leukoplakia.

Treatment. No treatment is required.

Congenital Lip Pits

Congenital lip pits represent a rare developmental malformation that may occur alone or in combination with commissural pits, cleft lip, or cleft palate. Clinically, they present as bilateral or unilateral depressions at the vermilion border of the lower lip (Fig. 5). A small amount of mucous secretion may accumulate at the depth of the pit. The lip may be enlarged and swollen.

Treatment of choice is surgical excision, but only for esthetic purposes.

Ankyloglossia

Ankyloglossia, or tongue-tie, is a rare developmental disturbance in which the lingual frenum is short or is attached close to the tip of the tongue (Fig. 6). In these cases the frenum is often thick and fibrous. Rarely, the condition may occur as a result of fusion between the tongue and the floor of the mouth or the alveolar mucosa. The malformation may cause speech difficulties.

Treatment. Surgical clipping of the frenum corrects the problem.

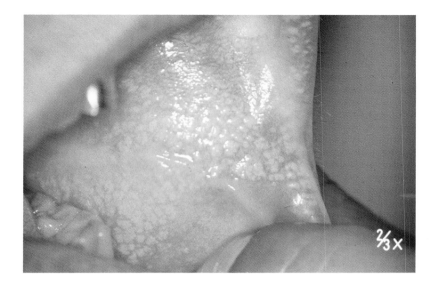

Fig. **4**. Fordyce's granules in the buccal mucosa.

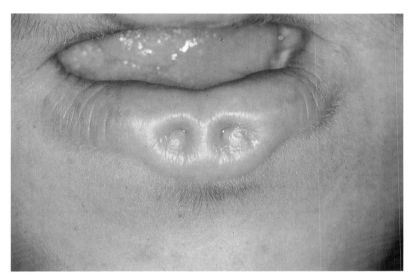

Fig. **5**. Congenital lip pits.

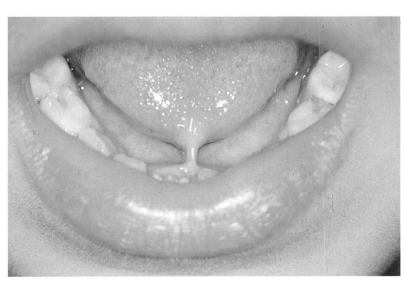

Fig. **6**. Ankyloglossia.

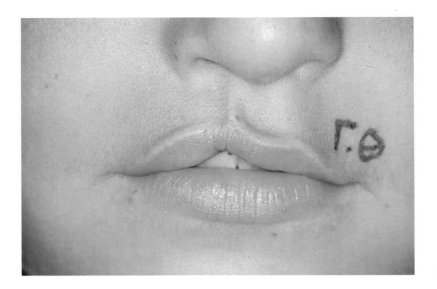

Fig. **7**. Cleft lip.

Cleft Lip

Cleft lip is a developmental malformation that usually involves the upper lip and very rarely the lower lip (Fig. **7**). It frequently coexists with cleft palate and it rarely occurs alone. The incidence of cleft lip alone or in combination with cleft palate varies from 0.52 to 1.34 per 1000 births.

The disorder may be unilateral or bilateral, complete or incomplete.

Treatment. Plastic surgery as early as possible corrects the esthetic and functional problems.

Cleft Palate

Cleft palate is a developmental malformation due to failure of the two embryonic palatal processes to fuse. The cause remains unknown, although heredity may play a role. Clinically, the patients exhibit a defect at the midline of the palate that may vary in severity (Fig. **8**). Bifid uvula represents a minor expression of cleft palate and may be seen alone or in combination with more severe malformations (Fig. **9**).

Cleft palate may occur alone or in combination with cleft lip. The incidence of cleft palate alone varies between 0.29 and 0.56 per 1000 births. It may occur in the hard or soft palate or both. Serious speech, feeding, and psychologic problems may occur.

Treatment. Early surgical correction is recommended.

Bifid Tongue

Bifid tongue is a rare developmental malformation that may appear in complete or incomplete form. The incomplete form is manifested as a deep furrow along the midline of the dorsum of the tongue or as a double ending of the tip of the tongue (Fig. **10**). Usually, it is an asymptomatic disorder requiring no therapy. It may coexist with the oro-facial digital syndrome.

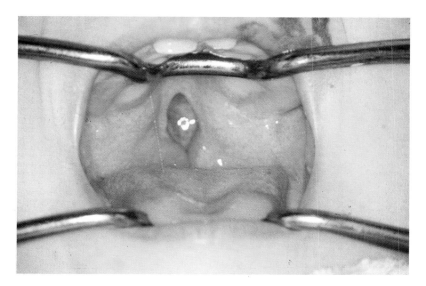

Fig. **8**. Cleft palate.

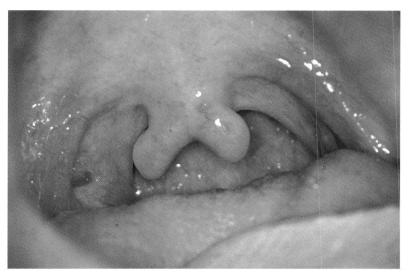

Fig. **9**. Bifid uvula.

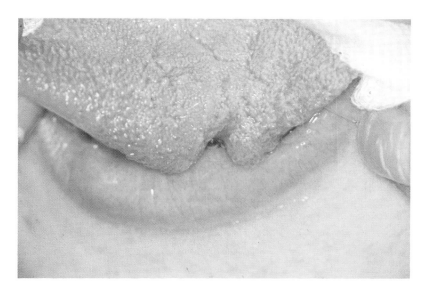

Fig. **10**. Bifid tongue.

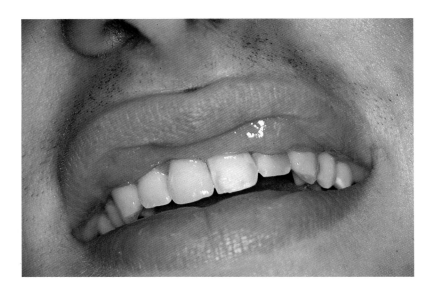

Fig. **11**. Double lip.

Double Lip

Double lip is a malformation characterized by a protruding horizontal fold of the inner surface of the upper lip (Fig. **11**). It may be congenital, but it can also occur as a result of trauma. The abnormality becomes prominent during speech or smiling. Frequently, it may be part of Ascher's syndrome.

Treatment. Surgical correction may be attempted for esthetic reasons only.

Torus Palatinus

Torus palatinus is a developmental malformation of unknown cause. It is a bony exostosis occurring along the midline of the hard palate. The incidence of torus palatinus is about 20% and appears in the third decade of life, but it also may occur at any age. The size of the exostosis varies, and the shape may be spindlelike, lobular, nodular, or even completely irregular (Fig. **12**). The exostosis is benign and consists of bony tissue covered with normal mucosa, although it may become ulcerated if traumatized. Because of its slow growth, the lesion causes no symptoms, and it is usually an incidental finding during physical examination.

Treatment. No treatment is needed, but problems may be anticipated if a total or partial denture is required.

Torus Mandibularis

Torus mandibularis is an exostosis covered with normal mucosa that appears on the lingual surfaces of the mandible, usually in the area adjacent to the bicuspids (Fig. **13**). The incidence of torus mandibularis is about 6%. Bilateral exostoses occur in 80% of the cases.

Clinically, it is an asymptomatic growth that varies in size and shape.

Treatment. Surgical removal of torus mandibularis is not indicated, but difficulties may be encountered if a denture has to be constructed.

Multiple Exostoses

Multiple exostoses are rare and may occur on the buccal surface of the maxilla. Clinically, they appear as multiple asymptomatic small nodular, bony elevations below the muccolabial fold covered with normal mucosa (Fig. **14**).

The cause is unknown and the lesions are benign, requiring no therapy.

Problems may be encountered during denture preparation.

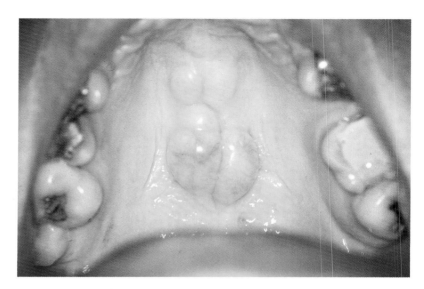

Fig. 12. Torus palatinus.

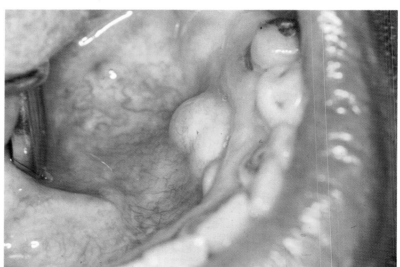

Fig. 13. Torus mandibularis.

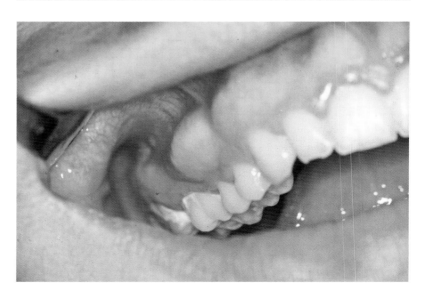

Fig. 14. Multiple exostoses.

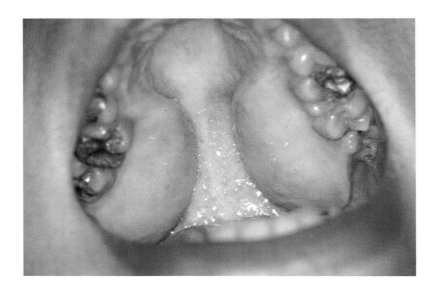

Fig. **15**. Fibrous developmental malformation of the maxillary tuberosities.

Fibrous Developmental Malformation

Fibrous developmental malformation is a rare developmental disorder consisting of fibrous overgrowth that usually occurs on the maxillary alveolar tuberosity. It appears as a bilateral symmetrical painless mass with a smooth surface, firm to palpation, and normal or pale color (Fig. **15**). Commonly, the malformation develops during the eruption of the teeth and may cover their crowns. The mass is firmly attached to the underlying bone but on occasion may be movable.

The classic sites of development are the maxillary alveolar tuberosity region, but rarely it may also appear in the retromolar region of the mandible and on the entire attached gingiva.

Treatment. Surgical excision is required if mechanical problems exist.

Facial Hemiatrophy

Facial hemiatrophy, or Parry-Romberg syndrome, is a developmental disorder of unknown cause characterized by unilateral atrophy of the facial tissues.

Sporadic hereditary cases have been described. The disorder becomes apparent in childhood and girls are affected more frequently than boys in a ratio of 3:2. In addition to facial hemiatrophy, epilepsy, trigeminal neuralgia, eye, hair, and sweat gland disorders may occur. The lipocytes on one side of the face disappear first, followed by skin, muscle, cartilage, and bone atrophy. Clini-

cally, the affected side appears atrophic and the skin is wrinkled and shriveled with hyperpigmentation occasionally (Fig. **16**).

Hemiatrophy of the tongue and the lips are the most common oral manifestations (Fig. **17**). Jaw and teeth disorders on the affected side may also occur.

The differential diagnosis includes true lipodystrophy, atrophy secondary to facial paralysis, facial hemihypertrophy, unilateral masseteric hypertrophy, and scleroderma.

Treatment is plastic reconstruction.

Masseteric Hypertrophy

Masseteric hypertrophy may be either congenital or functional as a result of an increased muscle function, bruxism, or habitual overuse of the masseters during mastication. The hypertrophy may be bilateral or unilateral. Clinically, masseteric hypertrophy appears as a swelling over the ascending ramus of the mandible, which characteristically becomes more prominent and firm when the patient clenches the teeth (Fig. **18**).

The differential diagnosis includes Sjögren's, Mikulicz's, and Heerfordt's syndromes, cellulitis, facial hemihypertrophy, and neoplasms.

Treatment. No treatment is necessary.

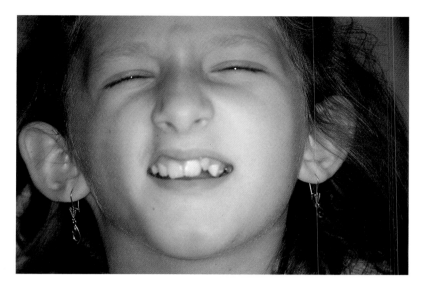

Fig. **16**. Hemiatrophy of the right side of the face.

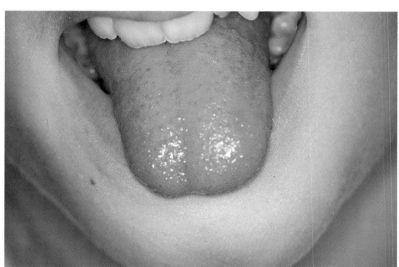

Fig. **17**. Atrophy of the right side of the tongue.

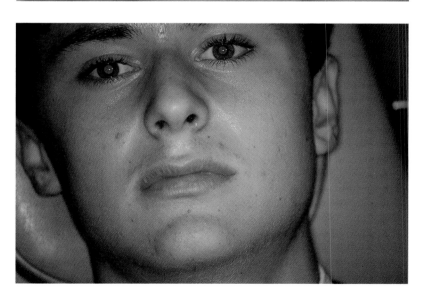

Fig. **18**. Hypertrophy of the left masseter.

3. Genetic Diseases

White Sponge Nevus

White sponge nevus, or Cannon's disease, is an uncommon disorder inherited as an autosomal dominant trait. It may appear at birth or more commonly during childhood. It is progressive until early adulthood, remaining stable thereafter. Clinically, the affected oral mucosa is white or gray-white with multiple furrows and a spongy texture (Fig. **19**). The lesions are benign, asymptomatic, and usually bilateral. Most frequently, they are found in the buccal mucosa and the ventral surface of the tongue but may occur anywhere in the mouth.

Some patients have similar lesions in the vaginal or rectal mucosa.

The differential diagnosis includes leukoplakia, lichen planus, leukoedema, pachyonychia congenita, congenital dyskeratosis, hereditary benign intraepithelial dyskeratosis, and mechanical whitish lesions.

Laboratory test. Histopathologic examination is helpful in establishing the diagnosis.

Treatment is not required.

Hereditary Benign Intraepithelial Dyskeratosis

Hereditary benign intraepithelial dyskeratosis is a genetic disorder inherited as an autosomal dominant trait with a high degree of penetrance. It affects the oral mucosa and the bulbar conjunctiva. The disease was first found in a triracial population (white, Indian, black) in North Carolina. Clinically, the oral lesions appear as thick, soft, white folds and plaques (Fig. **20**). They are firm and asymptomatic and the patient may not be aware of the lesions. Any region of the oral mucosa can be affected. The ocular lesion presents as a gelatinous plaque covering the pupil partially or totally and may cause temporary blindness. The plaque usually sheds and consequently vision is restored. This periodic appearance of the ocular lesion seems to show a seasonal pattern. The oral and conjunctival lesions appear usually during the first year of life.

The differential diagnosis includes white sponge nevus, dyskeratosis congenita, and rarely other genodermatoses associated with white hyperkeratotic lesions of the oral mucosa.

Laboratory tests. Histopathologic examination establishes the diagnosis.

Treatment. There is no need for treatment.

Gingival Fibromatosis

Gingival fibromatosis is transmitted as an autosomal dominant trait. It usually appears by the tenth year of life in both sexes. Clinically, there is generalized enlargement of the gingiva, which is usually firm, smooth, and occasionally nodular with minimal or no inflammation and normal or pale color (Fig. **21**).

The teeth may be partially or completely covered by the overgrown gingiva.

The upper gingivae are more severely affected and may prevent the eruption of the teeth.

The differential diagnosis should include gingival hyperplasia due to phenytoin and other drugs and gingival fibromatosis, which may occur as part of other genetic syndromes.

Treatment. Surgical excision of the enlarged gingiva.

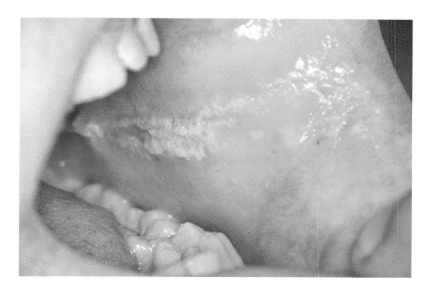

Fig. **19**. White sponge nevus of the buccal mucosa.

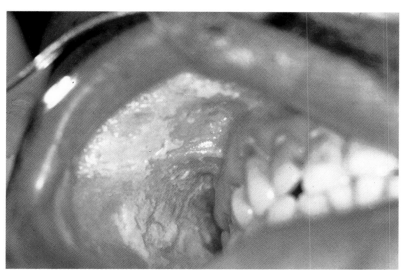

Fig. **20**. Hereditary benign intra-epithelial dyskeratosis, white lesions on the buccal mucosa.

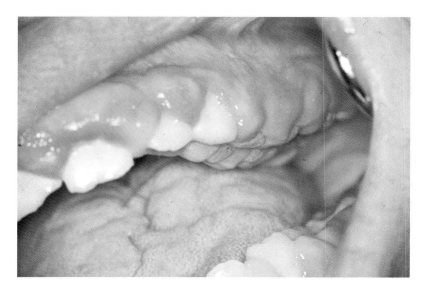

Fig. **21**. Gingival fibromatosis.

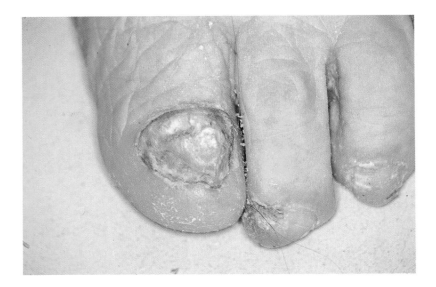

Fig. **22**. Pachyonychia congenita, thickening of the nails.

Pachyonychia Congenita

Pachyonychia congenita, or Jadassohn-Lewandowsky syndrome, is an autosomal dominant disease. It is characterized by symmetrical thickening of the nails (Fig. **22**), palmoplantar hyperkeratosis with hyperhidrosis, blister formation, follicular keratosis, and hyperkeratosis of the oral mucosa. The oral mucosal lesions are almost always present as thick and white or grayish-white areas that usually are located on the palate, dorsum of the tongue, and the buccal mucosa (Fig. **23**). These lesions appear at birth or shortly thereafter.

The differential diagnosis should include leukoplakia, lichen planus, white sponge nevus, dyskeratosis congenita, hereditary benign intraepithelial dyskeratosis, and focal palmoplantar and oral mucosa hyperkeratosis syndrome.

Treatment. No treatment is required.

Dyskeratosis Congenita

Dyskeratosis congenita, or Zinsser-Engman-Cole syndrome, is a disorder probably inherited as a recessive autosomal and X-linked trait. It is characterized by hyperpigmentation, telangiectasias, and atrophic areas of the skin (usually on the face, neck, and chest), dystrophic nails, hyperhidrosis, dermal and mucosal bullae, blepharitis (Fig. **24**), ectropion, aplastic anemia, mental handicap, and oral manifestations.

The oral lesions consist of aggregates or recurrent blisters that rupture, leaving a raw ulcerated surface mainly on the tongue and buccal mucosa. Atrophy of the oral mucosa is the result of repeated episodes. Finally, leukoplakia and squamous cell carcinoma may occur (Fig. **25**).

The differential diagnosis of the oral lesions should include leukoplakia, lichen planus, pachyonychia congenita, and epidermolysis bullosa.

Laboratory tests somewhat helpful for diagnosis are the blood cell examination and low serum gamma globulin levels.

Treatment is supportive.

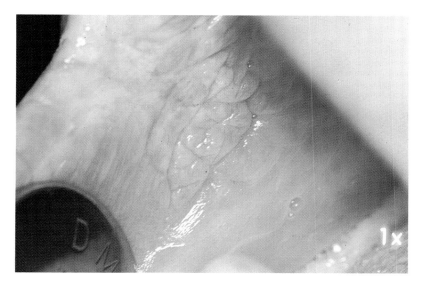

Fig. **23**. Pachyonychia congenita, grayish-white lesion on the buccal mucosa.

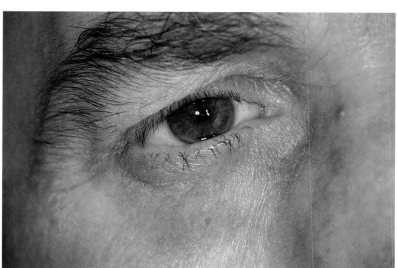

Fig. **24**. Dyskeratosis congenita, blepharitis.

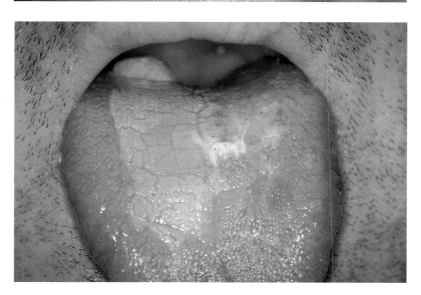

Fig. **25**. Dyskeratosis congenita, leukoplakia and verrucous carcinoma of the dorsal surface of the tongue.

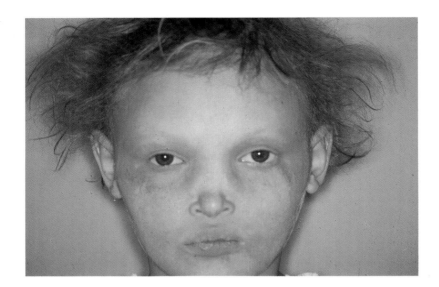

Fig. **26**. Hypohidrotic ectodermal dysplasia, characteristic face.

Hypohidrotic Ectodermal Dysplasia

Hypohidrotic ectodermal dysplasia is characterized by dysplastic changes of tissues of ectodermal origin and is usually inherited as an X-linked recessive trait, therefore affecting primarily males. The clinical hallmarks are characteristic facies with frontal bossing, large lips and ears, and a saddle nose (Fig. **26**); thin, dry skin and sparse, blond short hair, decreased sweating or complete anhidrosis, due to absence of sweat glands; absence of eyebrows; and oral lesions.

The characteristic finding in the oral cavity is hypodontia or anodontia (Fig. **27**). When teeth are present, they are hypoplastic and often have a conical shape. In some cases xerostomia may occur as a result of salivary gland hypoplasia. The disease usually presents during the first year of life, with a fever of unknown cause along with the retarded eruption or absence of the deciduous teeth.

The differential diagnosis includes idiopathic oligodontia, Papillon-Lefèvre syndrome, chondroectodermal dysplasia, cleidocranial dysplasia, and focal dermal hypoplasia.

Laboratory tests useful in establishing the diagnosis are dental radiographs and the demonstration of hypohidrosis or anhidrosis.

Treatment. There is no specific treatment. However, partial or full dentures must be contructed as early as possible.

Focal Palmoplantar and Oral Mucosa Hyperkeratosis Syndrome

Focal palmoplantar and oral mucosa hyperkeratosis syndrome is inherited as an autosomal dominant trait. It is also referred to as hyperkeratosis palmoplantaris and attached gingival hyperkeratosis and by many other names. The disorder is rare, characterized by focal hyperkeratosis at the weight-bearing and pressure-related areas of the palms, soles, and oral mucosa (Figs. **28, 29**). Marked hyperkeratosis of the attached gingiva is a constant finding (Fig. **30**). However, other areas bearing mechanical pressure or friction, such as the palate, alveolar mucosa, lateral border of the tongue, retromolar pad mucosa, and the buccal mucosa along the occlusal line may manifest hyperkeratosis, presenting clinically as leukoplakia. The hyperkeratosis appears early in childhood or at the time of puberty. The severity of the hyperkeratotic lesions increases with age and varies among patients, even in the same family. Rarely, hyperhidrosis, hyperkeratosis, and thickening of the nails may be observed.

The differential diagnosis should include pachyonychia congenita, dyskeratosis congenita, Papillon-Lefèvre syndrome, and oral leukoplakia and esophageal carcinoma syndrome.

Treatment. No reliably succesful treatment exists, but aromatic retinoids may occasionally be helpful.

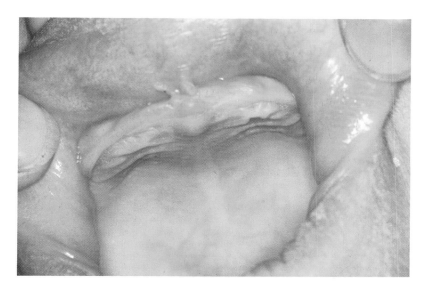

Fig. **27**. Hypohidrotic ectodermal dysplasia, anodontia.

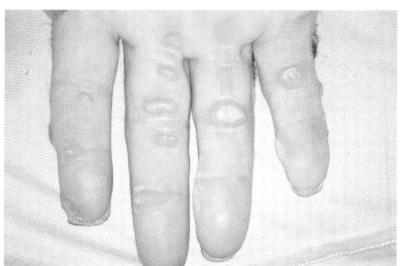

Fig. **28**. Focal palmoplantar and oral mucosa hyperkeratosis syndrome, hyperkeratosis of the palm.

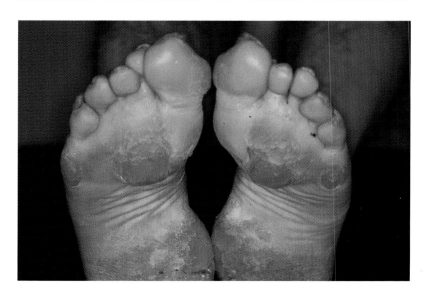

Fig. **29**. Focal palmoplantar and oral mucosa hyperkeratosis syndrome, hyperkeratosis of the soles.

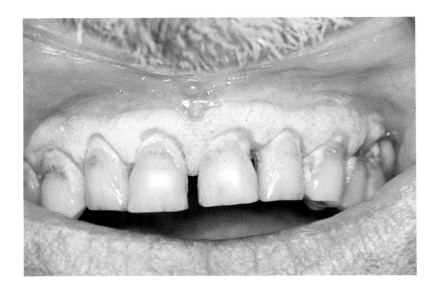

Fig. **30**. Focal palmoplantar and oral mucosa hyperkeratosis syndrome, hyperkeratosis of the attached gingiva.

Papillon-Lefèvre Syndrome

Papillon-Lefèvre syndrome is inherited as an autosomal recessive trait. It is characterized by hyperkeratosis of the palms and soles (Fig. **31**), severe destruction of periodontal tissues of both deciduous and permanent dentitions, and meningeal calcifications. Eruption of the deciduous teeth proceeds normally, but inflammation of the periodontal tissues, with periodontal pocket formation and bone destruction, ensues. The severe periodontitis results in premature loss of all the deciduous teeth by about the fourth year of age (Fig. **32**). The inflammatory response subsides at this stage and the gingiva resumes its normal appearance. The periodontitis again develops with the eruption of the permanent teeth and results in their loss. The oral mucosa appears normal even during the phase of active periodontal breakdown. The skin lesions usually appear between the second and fourth year of life and consist of well-demarcated, reddened and scaly hyperkeratosis of the palms and soles. Similar scaly red plaques may be seen on the dorsum of the fingers and toes, over the tibial tuberosity, and other areas of the skin.

The differential diagnosis should include juvenile periodontitis, histiocytosis X, acatalasia, hypophosphatemia, hypohidrotic ectodermal dysplasia, focal palmoplantar and oral mucosa hyperkeratosis syndrome, and other disorders that are associated with palmoplantar hyperkeratosis.

Treatment. Keratolytic agents and aromatic retinoids may help in the treatment of skin lesions. Therapy of the periodontal disease is always unsuccessful.

Benign Acanthosis Nigricans

Acanthosis nigricans is a rare disease involving the skin and mucosae, characterized by dark discoloration and papillary lesions. The disorder is classified into two major types: benign and malignant.

The benign variety is subdivided into: (1) genetic type that is manifested during childhood or early adolescence and rarely affects the oral cavity; (2) acanthosis nigricans that occurs as part of other syndromes, such as Prader-Willi, Crouzon, and Bloom syndromes, insulin-resistant diabetes mellitus, lupoid hepatitis, and hepatic cirrhosis; the syndromal type is manifested during childhood and does not involve the oral mucosa; and (3) pseudoacanthosis, which is an acquired form that affects obese and dark-skinned persons 25 to 60 years of age and involves the skin only.

Malignant acanthosis nigricans is an acquired form that is associated with a malignancy.

The genetic type of benign acanthosis nigricans involves the oral mucosa in about 10 to 15% of the cases. The tongue and lips are very often involved. Clinically, there is hypertrophy and elongation of the filliform papillae, resulting in a shaggy appearance of the tongue (Fig. **33**). The lips may be enlarged and covered by papillomatous growths, particularly at the commissures. The skin is thick with small velvety papillary lesions and dark pigmentation. The most common sites of involvement are the axillae, neck, groins, umbilicus, perianal area, and the genitalia.

The differential diagnosis includes hairy tongue and malignant acanthosis nigricans.

Laboratory test. Histopathologic findings are indicative but not specific.

Treatment. There is no treatment.

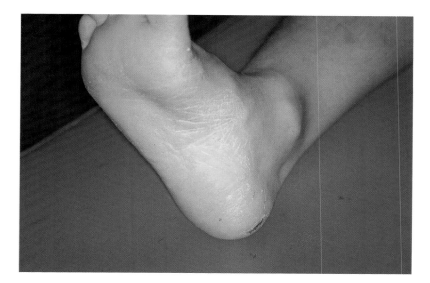

Fig. **31**. Papillon-Lefèvre syndrome, hyperkeratosis of the sole.

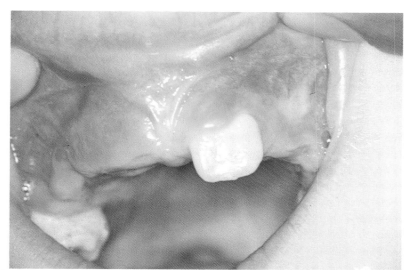

Fig. **32**. Papillon-Lefèvre syndrome, premature loss of deciduous teeth in a 6-year-old patient.

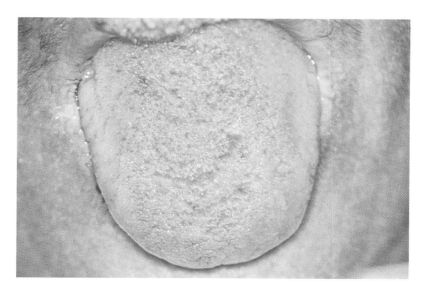

Fig. **33**. Benign acanthosis nigricans, hypertrophy and elongation of the filiform papillae of the tongue.

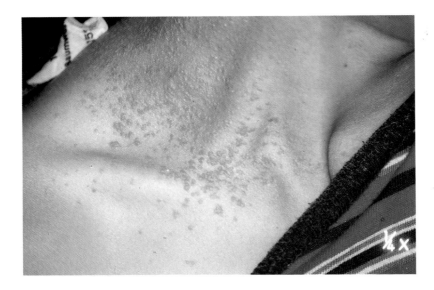

Fig. **34**. Dyskeratosis follicularis, multiple skin papules.

Dyskeratosis Follicularis

Dyskeratosis follicularis, or Darier-White disease, is an uncommon disorder inherited as an autosomal dominant trait.

It is more frequent in men and is manifested initially during childhood or early adolescence. The disease affects mainly the skin and nails, but the mucosae may also be involved (mouth, rectum, genitalia). The scalp, forehead, chest and back, ears, and nasolabial folds are usually affected.

Clinically, multiple skin papules that occasionally may coalesce into large plaques are seen (Fig. **34**). They are brownish-red in color and are covered by a yellowish to tan scaly crust. Hypertrophic and ulcerated lesions may also occur. The nails show subungual keratosis and longitudinal ridges and lines. The oral mucosa is affected in 20 to 40% of the cases, but the severity of oral lesions is independent of the activity of the disease in the skin.

The typical oral lesions are small whitish confluent papules, which may coalesce into plaques and become hypertrophic, assuming a cobblestone appearance (Fig. **35**). The palate, gingiva, buccal mucosa, and tongue are the most frequent sites of localization. The rectal, vaginal, vulval, and pharyngeal mucosae may also be involved.

The differential diagnosis includes acanthosis nigricans, papillary hyperplasia of the palate, warty dyskeratoma, and familial benign pemphigus.

Laboratory test. Histopathologic examination confirms the diagnosis.

Treatment. Vitamin A, retinoid acid, and salicylic acid are helpful.

Familial Benign Pemphigus

Familial benign pemphigus, or Hailey-Hailey disease, is a rare skin disease inherited as an autosomal dominant trait. Clinically, it is characterized by a recurrent group of small flaccid vesicles arising on an erythematous or normal skin base (Fig. **36**). The vesicles rapidly rupture, leaving erosions covered with crusts. The skin lesions are usually localized, with a tendency to spread peripherally, although the center heals with pigmentation or exhibits granular vegetations. Widespread lesions are unusual. The disease appears most frequently on the axillae, the groin, the neck, the perianal region, and the trunk.

The oral mucosa is rarely affected and always after the skin involvement. The oral lesions consist of groups of small vesicles that rupture easily, leaving denuded localized areas covered with pseudomembranes (Fig. **37**).

The disease usually begins between the second to third decade and has a good prognosis, although the clinical course is characterized by remissions and exacerbations and shows little tendency for improvement.

The differential diagnosis should include pemphigus, dyskeratosis follicularis, and rarely bullous and cicatricial pemphigoid and transient acantholytic dermatosis.

Laboratory test. Histopathologic examination supports the clinical diagnosis.

Treatment. Topical application of steroid and antifungal or antibacterial ointments or creams are of value in cases with secondary infection of the oral lesions. Systemic steroids are used only in severe cases.

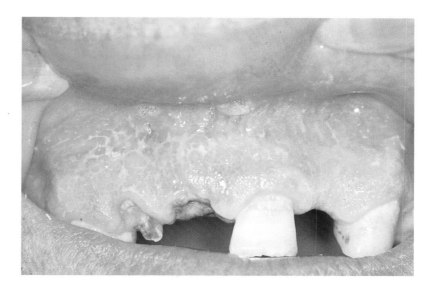

Fig. **35**. Dyskeratosis follicularis, multiple whitish confluent papules on the gingiva and alveolar mucosa.

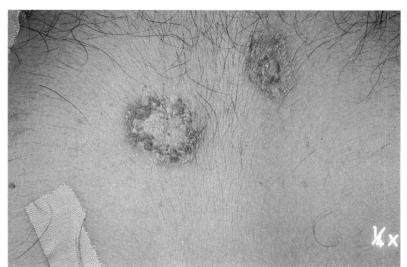

Fig. **36**. Familial benign pemphigus, skin lesions.

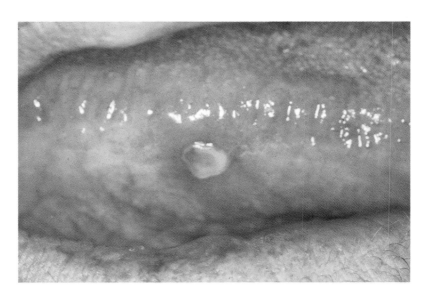

Fig. **37**. Familial benign pemphigus, erosion on the tongue.

Epidermolysis Bullosa

Epidermolysis bullosa is a group of inherited disorders characterized by bullae formation on the skin and mucous membranes spontaneously or after mechanical friction. Based on clinical, histopathologic, biochemical, ultrastructural, and genetic criteria the disorder falls into three major groups: nondystrophic, atrophic, and dystrophic.

In the nondystrophic subgroup is epidermolysis bullosa simplex, which includes several varieties. It is inherited as an autosomal dominant trait and begins at birth or early infancy. It is characterized by nonscarring generalized or localized bullae as a result of mechanical friction. The nails are spared. In the oral mucosa a few bullae may rarely occur, leaving erosions that heal without scarring (Fig. 38). The dentition is normal.

In the atrophic subgroup belong junctional epidermolysis bullosa, which is also called epidermolysis bullosa letalis, and generalized atrophic benign epidermolysis bullosa.

Both types are inherited as autosomal recessive traits. Lesions begin at birth or shortly after and consist of generalized bullae formation, which heals without scarring. The nails are involved. The oral mucosa shows bullae, severe ulcerations, and dysplastic teeth in the junctional type and mild lesions in the generalized atrophic benign type.

The prognosis is unfavorable for the first variety and good for the generalized atrophic benign type.

In the dystrophic subgroup belong dominant dystrophic epidermolysis bullosa and recessive dystrophic epidermolysis bullosa. Oral mucosal lesions are more common (about 50%) and severe in the recessive type. Clinically, bullae occur in areas of friction, which rupture leaving ulcers and scarring after the acute eruption. The tongue becomes depapillated and scarred (Fig. 39). Oral mucosal hyperplasia forming vegetating lesions, particularly on the palate, may be seen.

The teeth are usually dysplastic. Finally, leukoplakia, and squamous cell carcinomas may develop on the scars. The pharynx, larynx, esophagus, and anus are commonly affected. Generalized skin bullae leaving ulcerations that heal with scarring and milia formation are common in the recessive dystrophic type. The lesions are more often found on the hands, feet, knees, and elbows.

Dystrophy and loss of the nails are common (Fig. 40). In both types the lesions appear first at birth or infancy.

The prognosis is relatively good.

The differential diagnosis should include pemphigus, bullous pemphigoid, dermatitis herpetiformis, cicatricial pemphigoid of childhood, and bullous dermatoses of childhood.

Laboratory test. Histopathologic examination is important to establish the final diagnosis of different groups of epidermolysis bullosa.

Treatment. Therapy is nonspecific. Symptomatic topical therapy (antibiotics, steroids), systemic steroids, vitamin E, phenytoin, and retinoids have been used in severe cases.

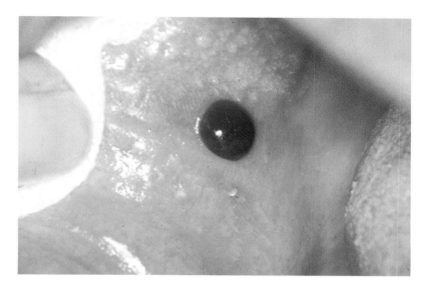

Fig. **38**. Epidermolysis bullosa simplex, hemorrhagic bulla on the buccal mucosa.

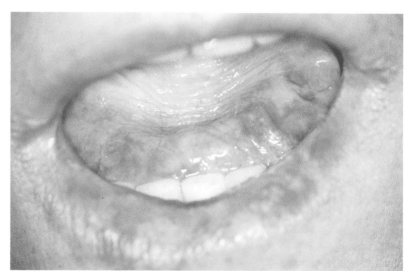

Fig. **39**. Epidermolysis bullosa, recessive dystrophic, depapillated and scarred tongue.

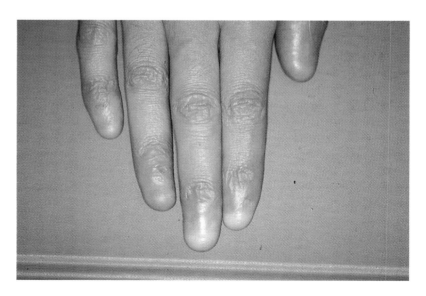

Fig. **40**. Epidermolysis bullosa, recessive dystrophic, dystrophy and loss of the fingernails.

Neurofibromatosis

Neurofibromatosis, or von Recklingshausen's disease, is a genetic disorder inherited as an autosomal dominant trait. The disease is characterized by café-au-lait spots (more than 6 spots over 1.5 cm in diameter are very suspicious of the disease), central nervous system manifestations, skeletal disorders, multiple neurofibromas, neurosarcomas in 3 to 12% of the cases, and endocrine disorders (such as pheochromocytoma).

The cardinal features of the disease are the café-au-lait spots and the skin neurofibromas. They usually appear during or after childhood. The skin neurofibromas are multiple and may be either cutaneous or subcutaneous (Fig. **41**). The oral cavity is uncommonly affected but may exhibit multiple or, rarely, isolated nodular neurofibromas, which vary in size (Fig. **42**).

The tongue, alveolar mucosa, and palate are the most commonly affected sites. Malignant transformation of oral neurofibromas is very rare. Involvement of the mandible and maxilla is also extremely rare.

The differential diagnosis should include multiple mucosal neuromas, multiple endocrine neoplasia type III syndrome, and the Klippel-Trenaunay-Weber syndrome.

Laboratory test. Histopathologic examination of oral and skin neurofibromas is helpful in establishing the diagnosis.

Treatment. Treatment is supportive and presents many problems for the dermatologist, surgeon, and endocrinologist.

Chondroectodermal Dysplasia

Chondroectodermal dysplasia, or Ellis-van Creveld syndrome, is inherited as an autosomal recessive trait. The main characteristics are bilateral polydactyly, chondrodysplasia of long bones, involvement of ectodermal tissues (hair, nails, teeth), and, rarely, congenital heart disease.

The most constant oral finding is fusion of the upper or lower lip to the gingiva, resulting in the disappearance of the mucolabial fold or multiple fibrous bands (Fig. **43**). Oligodontia and small conical teeth with enamel hypoplasia are also present.

The differential diagnosis includes oro-facial digital syndrome, acrofacial dysostosis of Weyers, other forms of chondrodystrophies.

Treatment is supportive.

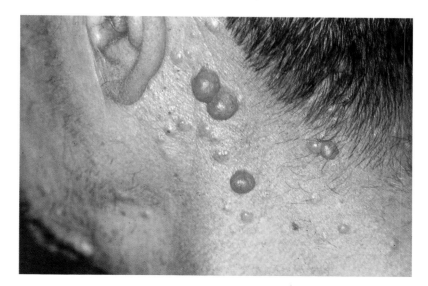

Fig. **41**. Neurofibromatosis, multiple cutaneous neurofibromas.

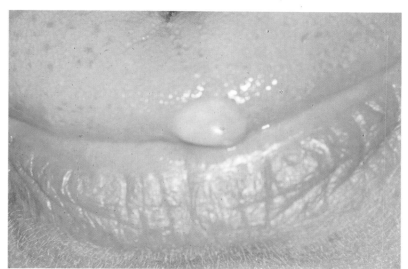

Fig. **42**. Neurofibromatosis, solitary neurofibroma of the tongue.

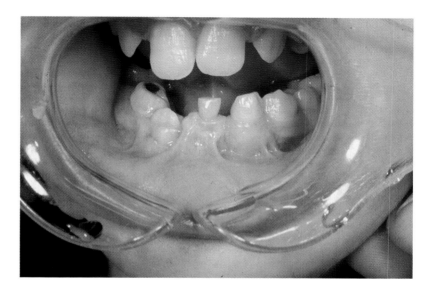

Fig. **43**. Chondroectodermal dysplasia, disappearance of the mucolabial sulcus and multiple fibrous bands.

Hereditary Hemorrhagic Telangiectasia

Hereditary hemorrhagic telangiectasia or Osler-Rendu-Weber disease is inherited as an autosomal dominant trait.

Characterized by dysplasia of the capillaries and small vessels, the disease usually develops during adolescence and affects both sexes. The cardinal manifestations are mucosal, cutaneous, and internal organ (liver, spleen, stomach) telangiectases. Morphologically, three varieties of telangiectases have been described: microscopic lesions of less than a millimeter in diameter, nodules, and spiderlike lesions.

These lesions have a bright red, purple, or violet color and disappear on pressure with a glass slide. The oral mucosa is frequently involved with multiple lesions on the lip and the dorsum of the tongue (Fig. 44). The palate, buccal mucosa, and gingiva may be less frequently involved. Hemorrhage from oral lesions is frequent after minimal mechanical damage, such as tooth brushing.

Epistaxis and gastrointestinal bleeding are early, common, and occasionally serious complications.

The differential diagnosis includes varicosities of the tongue, Maffucci's syndrome, and Fabry's disease.

Laboratory test. Histopathologic examination confirms the clinical diagnosis.

Treatment. Control of spontaneous hemorrhage. The angiomatous lesions may sometimes be excised surgically, cauterized, or treated with the cryoprobe.

Peutz-Jeghers Syndrome

Peutz-Jeghers syndrome is transmitted as an autosomal dominant disorder with a high degree of penetrance, characterized by intestinal polyposis and mucocutaneous pigmented spots. The manifestations, which may be apparent at any age, include intestinal polyps (hamartomas) 0.5 to 7 cm in diameter and pigmented spots. About 50% of the patients have numerous dark spots on the perioral skin, the nose, and around the eyes. Similar spots may occur in other regions.

Pigmented spots 1 to 10 mm in diameter are always found in the oral mucosa, particularly on the lower lip and the buccal mucosa, but rarely on the upper lip, the tongue, the palate, and the gingiva (Fig. 45). Oral pigmentation constitutes the most important diagnostic finding and appears in the form of oval, round, or irregular brown or black spots or patches.

The differential diagnosis includes Addison's disease, Albright's syndrome, simple freckles, and normal pigmentation.

Laboratory test. Radiologic evaluation of the gastrointestinal tract is helpful in establishing the diagnosis.

Treatment. Supportive treatment of gastrointestinal bleeding.

Maffucci's Syndrome

Maffucci's syndrome is a rare disease of uncertain cause. It is not clear whether it represents an inherited disorder or a dysplasia. Both sexes may be affected. Clinical characteristics include multiple enchondromas, principally in the small bones of the hands and feet, although any bone of cartilaginous origin may be affected; multiple hemangiomas localized on the skin, mucosae, and viscera; phleboliths; and pigmented skin macules. The oral mucosa is rarely affected and the oral lesions usually are multiple hemangiomas. The tongue is the most frequent site of hemangiomas, but the buccal mucosa, lips, soft palate, and other oral regions can also be involved (Fig. 46). In a recent review only 8 of 110 cases were found to have oral hemangiomas.

Chondrosarcomas, hemangiosarcomas, and multiple fractures may be the most severe complications of the disease.

The diagnosis should be based on clinical and histopathologic evidence.

The differential diagnosis includes hemangiomas, Ollier's disease, the blue rubber bleb nevus syndrome, and the Klippel-Trenaunay-Weber syndrome.

Laboratory tests. Histopathologic and radiographic examinations confirm the diagnosis.

Treatment. Surgical excision of the enchondromas and hemangiomas may be attempted if they are symptomatic.

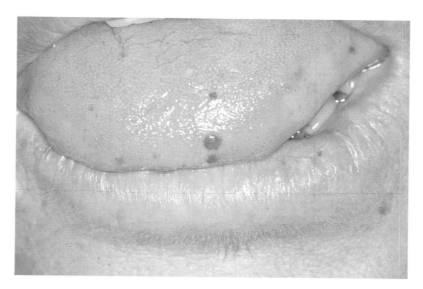

Fig. **44**. Hereditary hemorrhagic telangiectasia, multiple lesions on the tongue.

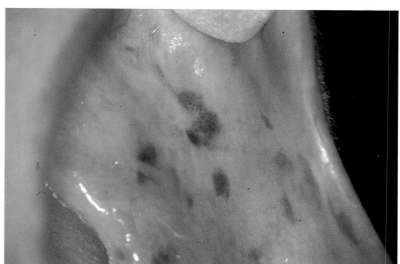

Fig. **45**. Peutz-Jeghers syndrome, multiple pigmented spots on the buccal mucosa.

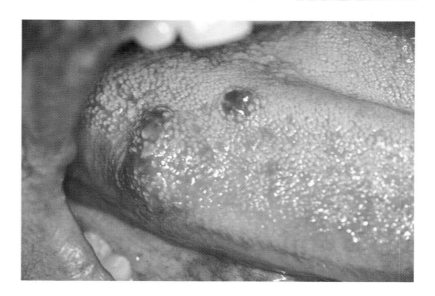

Fig. **46**. Maffucci's syndrome, multiple hemangiomas of the tongue.

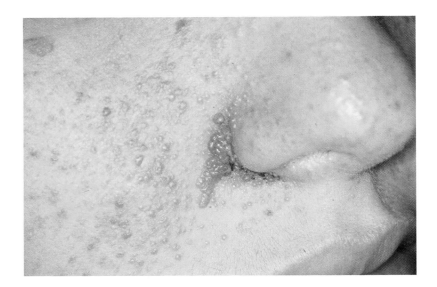

Fig. **47**. Tuberous sclerosis, numerous facial angiofibromas (adenoma sebaceum).

Tuberous Sclerosis

Tuberous sclerosis, or Bourneville-Pringle syndrome, is transmitted as an autosomal dominant trait. It is characterized by epilepsy, mental handicap, paraventricular calcifications, multiple small gliomas, mucocutaneous manifestations, skeletal disorders, and, rarely, ophthalmic tumors. The disease affects equally both sexes and usually presents between the ages of 2 and 6 years. Many patients die by the age of 20 years.

Characteristic lesions occur on the face, principally along the nasolabial fold and cheeks. These are numerous small nodules, red to pink in color, which are actually angiofibromas, although the prevailing term is "adenoma sebaceum" (Fig. **47**). Other cutaneous changes are white macules (maple leaf or ash leaf), café-au-lait spots, skin tags, and multiple periungual fibromas. The oral mucosa may be involved in about 10% of the cases. The gingiva or other parts of the oral mucosa may exhibit confluent nodules a few millimeters to less than 1 cm in diameter, which are of whitish or normal color (Fig. **48**). Enamel hypoplasia may also occur.

The differential diagnosis of oral lesions should include multiple fibromas, multiple condylomata acuminata, focal epithelial hyperplasia, and neurofibromatosis.

Laboratory test. Histophatologic examination of skin and oral mucosa lesions and skull radiographs are helpful in the diagnosis. The epilepsy should be evaluated by electroencephalography.

Treatment. There is no specific therapy, but anticonvulsive drugs may be required.

Sturge-Weber Syndrome

Sturge-Weber syndrome is a sporadic congenital dysplasia. Both sexes may be affected. It is characterized by hemangiomas of the face and oral mucosa, and of the leptomeninges, calcification of the brain, ocular disorders, epilepsy, and mild mental handicap.

The facial hemangioma is the most constant finding and is apparent at birth. It is unilateral, has a bright red or purple color, and is confined roughly to the area supplied by the trigeminal nerve (Fig. **49**). Hemangiomas of the oral mucosa are unilateral, rarely cross the midline, and may involve the upper gingiva, buccal mucosa, lips, and tongue (Fig. **50**). These lesions have a bright red or purple color and are usually flat but may also have a raised irregular surface that causes tissue enlargement. The ipsilateral permanent teeth may erupt early and may be ectopic, although delayed tooth eruption may also occur. Care must be taken during tooth extractions because hemorrhage may be severe. When the classic signs and symptoms are present, the diagnosis of Sturge-Weber syndrome is apparent.

The differential diagnosis includes large disseminated hemangiomas and the Klippel-Trenaunay-Weber syndrome.

Laboratory tests helpful in diagnosis and management are angiography, electroencephalography, skull radiographs and computed tomography.

Treatment. The therapy is guided by the symptoms and is supportive.

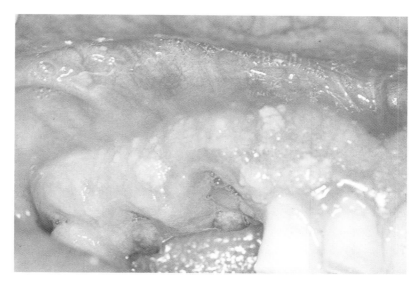

Fig. **48**. Tuberous sclerosis, confluent whitish nodules on the gingiva and the alveolar mucosa.

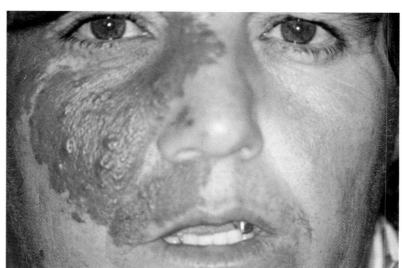

Fig. **49**. Sturge-Weber syndrome, facial hemangioma.

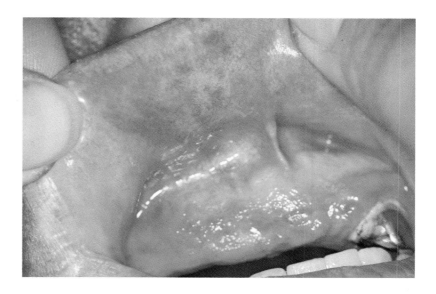

Fig. **50**. Sturge-Weber syndrome, oral hemangioma.

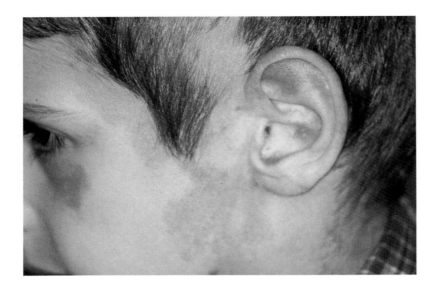

Fig. **51**. Klippel-Trenaunay-Weber syndrome, facial hemangiomas.

Klippel-Trenaunay-Weber Syndrome

Klippel-Trenaunay-Weber syndrome, or angio-osteohypertrophy, is a rare dysplastic vascular disorder. It is characterized by multiple facial hemangiomas (Fig. **51**), vascular masses that involve soft tissues and bone and are accompanied by asymmetric enlargement of the extremities, vascular cutaneous lesions, ocular disorders (scleral pigmentation, cataract, glaucoma, and iris heterochromia) (Fig. **52**), hemangiomas in internal organs, and oral hemangiomas. Clinically, the oral hemangiomas are usually located on the soft and hard palates and gingiva, which may be enlarged (Fig. **53**). Premature tooth eruption and bony overgrowth may produce malocclusion.

The differential diagnosis includes Sturge-Weber syndrome, Maffucci's syndrome, and large isolated hemangiomas.

Treatment is supportive.

Cowden's Disease

Cowden's disease is an autosomal dominant disorder characterized by multiple hamartomas and cancers of the breast, thyroid, and other organs. The cutaneous manifestations are multiple hamartomatous papules, and nodules.

Oral lesions consist of small whitish papules or nodules that may be isolated or coalesce in a cobblestone pattern, usually on the gingiva (Fig. **54**).

The differential diagnosis includes tuberous sclerosis, multiple mucosal neuromas, endocrine neoplasia type III syndrome, and malignant acanthosis nigricans.

Laboratory test. Histopathologic examination is helpful in establishing the diagnosis.

Treatment. No treatment is available.

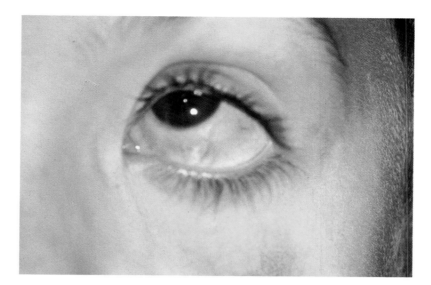

Fig. **52**. Klippel-Trenaunay-Weber syndrome, ocular pigmentation.

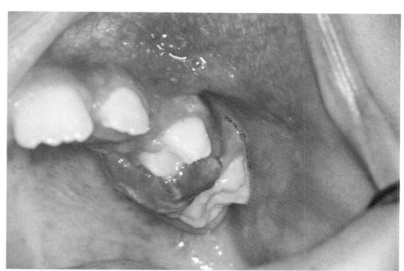

Fig. **53**. Klippel-Trenaunay-Weber syndroma, oral hemangiomas.

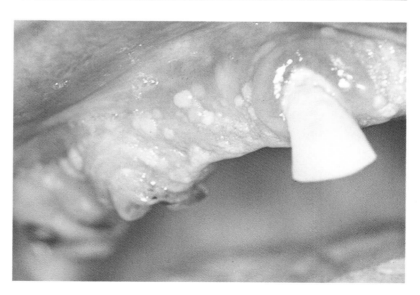

Fig. **54**. Cowden's disease, multiple whitish nodules on the alveolar mucosa.

Cleidocranial Dysplasia

Cleidocranial dysplasia is transmitted as an autosomal dominant trait. It is characterized by unilateral or bilateral hypoplasia or complete absence of the clavicles (as a result the patient has the capability of approximating his or her shoulders (Fig. 55), skull abnormalities (delayed closure or open fontanelles, open sutures, large skull, broad flat nose), exophthalmos, deafness, and oral lesions. The oral manifestations consist of a high, narrow angulated palate, delayed eruption or noneruption of the deciduous and permanent teeth, and supernumerary unerupted permanent teeth (Fig. 56). The teeth may be malformed. Periodontal disease is commonly found.

The differential diagnosis includes hypohidrotic ectodermal dysplasia, focal dermal hypoplasia, craniofacial dysostosis, and Apert's syndrome.

Laboratory test. Radiographic examination is helpful for the diagnosis.

Treatment. No treatment is available. Dental care is essential.

Oro-Facial Digital Syndrome

Oro-facial digital syndrome type I is a rare X-linked dominant inherited disorder lethal to males. The oro-facial digital syndrome type II is inherited as an autosomal recessive trait.

The cardinal clinical manifestations of syndrome type I are digital malformations (brachydactyly, syndactyly, clinodactyly) and other skeletal disorders, cutaneous lesions (milia, xeroderma, alopecia, sparse hair, dermatoglyphic abnormalities), mental handicap, ocular hypertelorism, and oral lesions, which are numerous and variable. Constant oral mucosal findings are the multiple hyperplastic frenula traversing the upper and lower gingivolabial folds (Fig. 57). There is also hypertrophy and shortening of the frenula of upper and lower lips and tongue.

The tongue is multilobed or bifid and often exhibits multiple hamartomas. Clefts of the lips and the soft and hard palates are common. Mandibular lateral incisors are often missing, supernumerary teeth are common, and upper canine are malpositioned.

The differential diagnosis should include oro-facial digital syndrome type II (Mohr syndrome), chondroectodermal dysplasia, and oculodentodigital syndrome.

Treatment. No treatment is available, but the oral problem requires dental care.

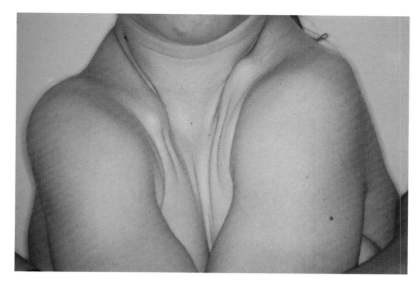

Fig. **55**. Cleidocranial dysplasia, hypermobility of the shoulder.

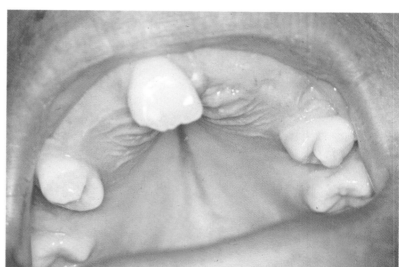

Fig. **56**. Cleidocranial dysplasia, high palate and noneruption of some permanent teeth.

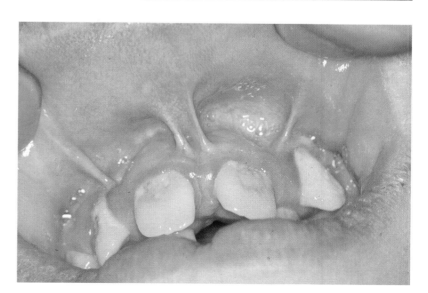

Fig. **57**. Oro-facial digital syndrome, multiple hyperplastic frenula.

Focal Dermal Hypoplasia

The focal dermal hypoplasia, or Goltz syndrome, is a rare disorder that affects females almost exclusively. The mode of inheritance is not clearly known; probably a single gene mode of inheritance is involved. The syndrome is characterized by irregular linear skin pigmentation, atrophy, and telangiectasia present at birth, localized deposits of subcutaneous fat that present as soft reddish-yellow nodules (Fig. **58**), syndactyly, especially between the third and fourth fingers, polydactyly, dystrophic nails, sparse hair, skeletal malformations, occasionally mental handicap, and mucous membrane involvement.

The oral mucosal manifestations are multiple papillomas on the tongue (Fig. **59**), buccal mucosa, palate, gingiva, or lips. Similar papillomatous lesions may occur on the vulva, perianal, and perioral areas. Oligodontia, small teeth, dysplastic enamel, and malocclusion are not rare. The diagnosis is made on clinical criteria.

The differential diagnosis of oral lesions should include multiple papillomas and condylomata acuminata, focal epithelial hyperplasia, and incontinentia pigmenti.

Laboratory test. Histopathologic examination is essential to confirm oral papilloma and the fatty collections in the skin nodules.

Treatment is supportive. Surgical excision of oral papillomas.

Incontinentia Pigmenti

Incontinentia pigmenti is a disease inherited as an X-linked dominant trait that is lethal in males. The lesions usually appear at birth or within the first month as vesiculobullous eruptions in a linear group usually scattered on the trunk and perimammary regions or on the extremities, papuloverrucous irregular linear lesions of the skin, characteristic skin pigmentation, which may be the only abnormality (Fig. **60**), other disorders (alopecia, dystrophic nails, ocular defects, skeletal and neurologic abnormalities), and dental defects, which include impacted teeth, dysplastic enamel, peg-shaped or conical teeth, delayed dentition, and oligodontia (Fig. **61**).

The differential diagnosis should include epidermolysis bullosa, congenital syphilis, hypohidrotic ectodermal dysplasia, and focal dermal hypoplasia.

Laboratory test. Histopathologic examination is useful in establishing the diagnosis.

Treatment. No treatment is available.

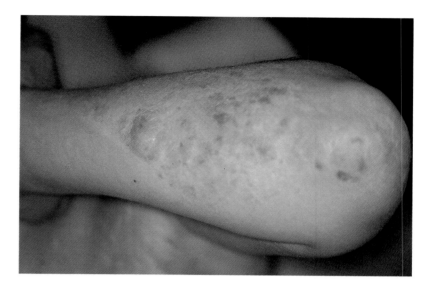

Fig. **58**. Focal dermal hypoplasia, multiple localized nodules on the skin.

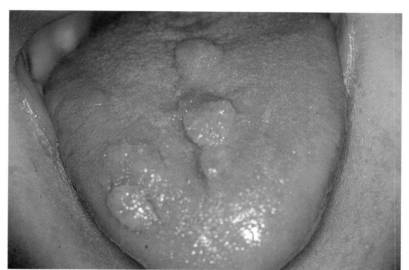

Fig. **59**. Focal dermal hypoplasia, multiple papillomas on the tongue.

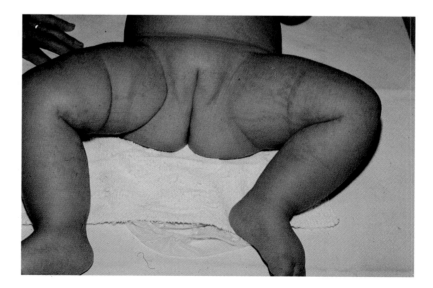

Fig. **60**. Incontinentia pigmenti, dirty brown hyperpigmentation of the skin.

Ehlers-Danlos Syndrome

Ehlers-Danlos syndrome is a group of disorders inherited as an autosomal dominant, autosomal recessive, or X-linked recessive trait. On the basis of genetic, clinical, and biochemical criteria, at least 11 types of Ehlers-Danlos syndrome are now recognized. Although the basic defect is not well known, an abnormality in collagen biosynthesis has been recorded in some of the subgroups.

The cardinal clinical features of the syndrome are hyperextensibility of the skin, hyperextensibility of joints, cutaneous fragility, bruisability, and pseudotumors, fragility of blood vessels and delayed wound healing, ocular abnormalities, and oral manifestations.

The oral mucosa is excessively fragile and subject to bruising. Gingival bleeding and periodontitis are common. Wound healing may be only slightly delayed. Tooth mobility is not increased, although a hypermobility of the temporomandibular joint may occur. Approximately 50% of patients have the ability to touch their nose with the tongue tip compared with 10% of normal persons (Fig. **62**). Dental abnormalities, such as enamel, dentine, and cementum defects and an increased tendency to develop multiple pulp stones, have been reported.

The differential diagnosis includes cutis laxa, Marfan's syndrome and Marfanoid hypermobility syndrome, and osteogenesis imperfecta.

Laboratory tests, such as histopathologic and blood examinations are suggestive but not diagnostic.

Treatment. There is no definitive treatment for the syndrome. Supportive measures against skin fragility, trauma, etc., should be included in the management of patients.

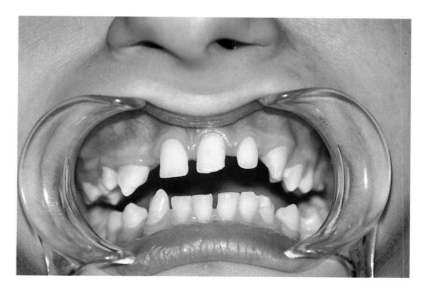

Fig. **61**. Incontinentia pigmenti, oligodontia and peg-shaped teeth.

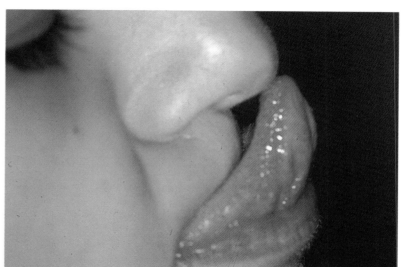

Fig. **62**. Ehlers-Danlos syndrome, ability to touch the tip of the nose with the tongue tip.

4. Mechanical Injuries

Traumatic Ulcer

Traumatic ulcers are common oral lesions. The causes are variable and include a sharp or broken tooth, rough fillings, clumsy use of cutting dental instruments, hard foodstuffs, sharp foreign bodies, biting of the mucosa, and denture irritation. Ulcers of traumatic origin may occur anywhere in the mouth but are most commonly found on the lateral borders of the tongue (Figs. **63, 64**), the buccal mucosa, the lips (Fig. **65**), the labioalveolar and buccalveolar grooves (Fig. **66**).

The size of the ulcer may vary from a few millimeters to several centimeters in diameter and depends on the intensity, duration, and type of the trauma as well as superimposed infection.

The clinical presentation is variable, but usually traumatic ulcers appear as single painful lesions with a smooth red or white-yellow surface and thin erythematous margins. They are usually soft to palpation and heal without scarring within 6 to 10 days, spontaneously or after removal of the cause.

However, when the cause is sustained and intense, the ulcer surface may become irregular with vegetations, the border may become raised, and the base indurated. In these cases the traumatic ulcer may clinically resemble a carcinoma.

Subjective complaints vary from mild to severe, depending on the depth and location of the ulcer in the mouth. The diagnosis is based on the history and clinical features. Once a relationship has been established between an ulcerogenic factor and an ulcer, removal of the cause is mandatory, with follow-up of the patient for 7 to 10 days to verify complete healing. If the ulcer persists, then revision of the clinical diagnosis and performance of a biopsy to rule out cancer is recommended.

The differential diagnosis should include squamous cell carcinoma and other cancers, syphilis, tuberculosis, aphthae, and eosinophilic and other ulcers.

Laboratory test. Histopathologic examination often helps in establishing the diagnosis.

Treatment. Removal of the traumatic factors.

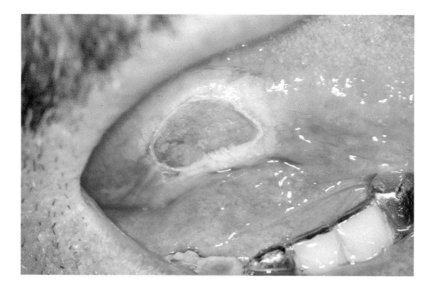

Fig. **63**. Traumatic ulcer of the tongue.

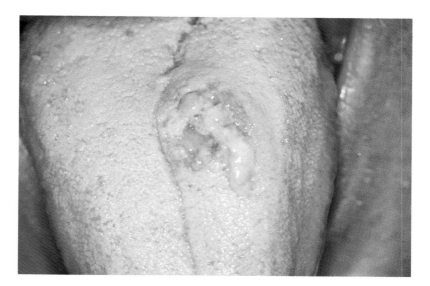

Fig. **64**. Traumatic ulcer of the tongue.

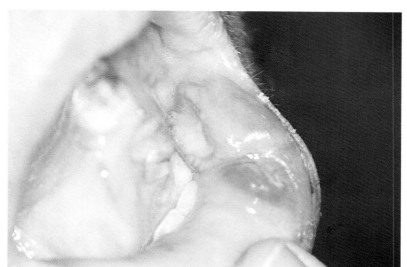

Fig. **65**. Traumatic ulcer on the lower lip.

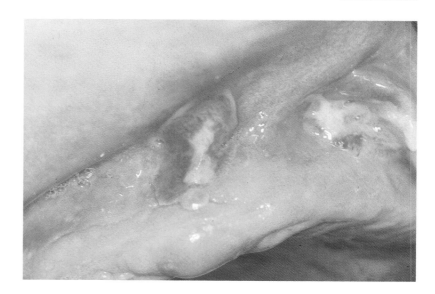

Fig. **66**. Traumatic ulcer on the labioalveolar groove caused by dentures.

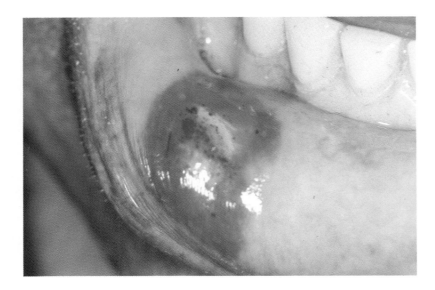

Fig. **67**. Traumatic hematoma on the lower lip.

Traumatic Hematoma

Traumatic hematoma of the oral mucosa occurs under the influence of mild or severe mechanical forces that result in hemorrhage within the oral tissues. Clinically, it appears as an irregular lesion with a deep red hue (Fig. **67**). The most common sites of hematoma are the tongue and lips and the most common causes are biting of the oral mucosa or careless use of dental instruments.

Chronic Biting

Mild chronic biting of the oral mucosa is common in anxious persons. These patients consciously bite the buccal mucosa, tongue, or lips and tear off the superficial epithelial layers. Clinically, this lesion is characterized by a diffuse irregular area of small furrows, whitish surface, and desquamation of the affected epithelium (Fig. **68**). Infrequently, there are surface erosions and petechiae.

The differential diagnosis includes leukoedema, Fordyce's granules, candidosis, leukoplakia, white sponge nevus, and lichen planus.

Treatment includes mild sedatives and warning the patient about the deleterious results of this habit on the oral mucosa.

Toothbrush Trauma

Toothbrush trauma may occur during aggressive tooth-brushing with a hard brush. The clinical picture consists of small oval, round, or bandlike superficial erosions located on the gingiva and alveolar mucosa (Fig. **69**). These lesions cause mild subjective complaints and heal rapidly.

The differential diagnosis includes herpes simplex, aphthous ulcers and other traumatic lesions.

Factitious Trauma

Patients mentally handicapped or with serious emotional problems may resort to oral self-inflicted trauma.

The trauma is usually inflicted through biting, fingernails, or through the use of a sharp object.

These lesions are slow to heal due to perpetuation of the injury by the patient. The most frequent locations are the tongue, the lower lip, and the gingiva (Fig. **70**).

The diagnosis depends on strong clinical suspicion and the history, although many patients deny that they are responsible for the observed traumatic lesions.

The differential diagnosis includes traumatic ulcer, malignant ulcer, tuberculosis, syphilis, and aphthous ulcer.

Treatment should include local measures and psychiatric therapy, if appropriate.

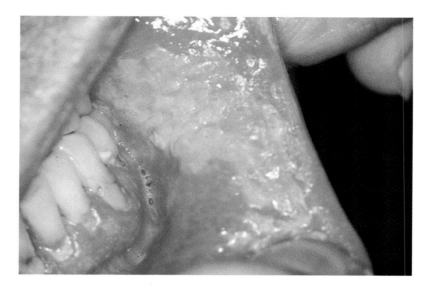

Fig. **68**. Chronic biting of the buccal mucosa.

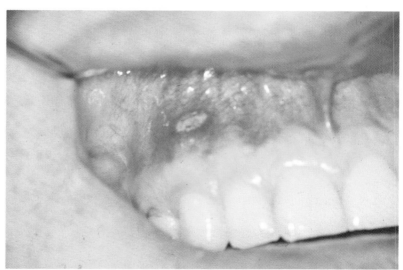

Fig. **69**. Erosion caused by tooth-brushing.

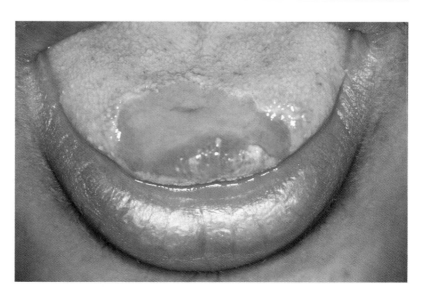

Fig. **70**. Factitious ulcer on the tongue.

Fellatio

Apart from venereal diseases, oral lesions may occur due to negative pressure or mechanical irritation applied during fellatio. Lesions occur at the junction of the soft and hard palate and consist of petechiae, erythema, and ecchymoses (Fig. **71**). They disappear spontaneously within a week.

The differential diagnosis includes traumatic injury, infectious mononucleosis, thrombocytopenic purpura, leukemia, and aplastic anemia.

Lingual Frenum Ulcer After Cunnilingus

Traumatic oral erosion or ulcer may result from practice of orogenital sex. Lingual frenum ulcer secondary to cunnilingus may be seen particularly in males. The lesion develops as the taut lingual frenum is rubbed over the rough incisal edges of the mandibular incisors during the tongue movements in cunnilingus. Clinically, the lesion is characterized by a small nonspecific erosion or ulcer covered by a whitish exudate and surrounded by a red halo (Fig. **72**).

The differential diagnosis should include other traumatic erosions or ulcers, primary and secondary syphilis, minor aphthous ulcer, and secondary herpetic lesions.

Cotton Roll Stomatitis

Cotton rolls are applied in dental practice to keep the dental surfaces dry. Excessive drying of the mucosal surfaces may result in erosions during rough removal of the cotton, which adheres to the mucosa. Clinically, the lesions appear as painful erosions covered with a whitish pseudomembrane, and they heal within 4 to 6 days (Fig. **73**).

The differential diagnosis includes other traumatic or chemically induced lesions and aphthous ulcers.

Treatment. No treatment is necessary.

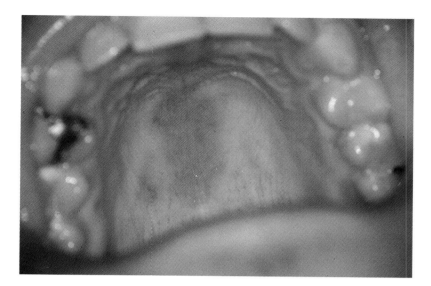

Fig. **71**. Erythema on the palate caused by fellatio.

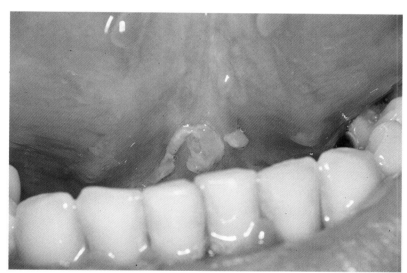

Fig. **72**. Lingual frenum ulcer after cunnilingus.

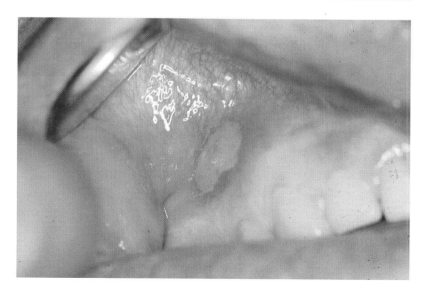

Fig. **73**. Erosion caused by cotton roll.

Denture Stomatitis

Denture stomatitis or denture sore mouth is frequent in patients who wear dentures for long periods of time. Usually, the lesion is confined to the maxilla and only rarely occurs on the mandibular mucosal surface. Clinically, the mucosa beneath the denture is edematous, red with or without whitish spots that represent accumulation of hyphae of Candida albicans, or food remnants (Fig. 74). The mucosal surface is smooth or granular.

Most patients are asymptomatic but some complain of a burning sensation or irritation and pain. The lesions are benign and may be localized or generalized. The most important causative factors of denture stomatitis are trauma from the denture, food debris accumulating under the denture surface, and C. albicans infection.

The differential diagnosis includes allergic contact stomatitis due to acrylic.

Treatment. Improvement of denture fit, good oral hygiene, and nystatin or clotrimazole if C. albicans is present.

Epulis Fissuratum

Epulis fissuratum, or denture fibrous hyperplasia is a common tissue reaction caused by poorly fitting dentures in persons who have been wearing dentures for a long period of time. The chronic irritation may be due to a sharp margin of the denture or overextended flanges. The lesion presents as multiple or single inflamed elongated mucosal papillary folds in the mucolabial or mucobuccal grooves (Fig. 75).

These hyperplastic folds are mobile, somewhat firm to palpation, and their continued growth may cause problems in maintaining denture retention. Painful ulceration is common in the base of the fold.

The differential diagnosis includes multiple fibromas, neurofibromatosis, and squamous cell carcinoma.

Treatment. Surgical excision of the hyperplastic folds and new denture construction.

Papillary Hyperplasia of the Palate

Papillary hyperplasia of the palate is a variety of denture stomatitis occurring in patients who wear ill-fitting dentures for many years.

However, similar lesions may occur in edentulous persons with high arched palate due to mechanical irritation of foodstuffs on the palate. Clinically, the lesions appear as multiple coalescing small edematous, reddish elevations that usually measure 1 to 2 mm or more in diameter (Fig. 76). The lesions are confluent and occupy part or all of the hard palate, giving it a cauliflower-like appearance. These lesions are asymptomatic as a rule and may be accidentally discovered by the patient, who becomes anxious, fearing a cancer. They are benign and should not be a cause for alarm.

The differential diagnosis includes acanthosis nigricans, multiple condylomata acuminata, dyskeratosis follicularis, and tuberculosis.

Treatment consists of reassurance of the patient regarding the nature of the lesion. These lesions should be removed before the construction of a new denture.

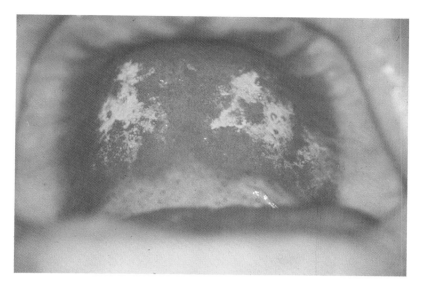

Fig. **74**. Denture stomatitis.

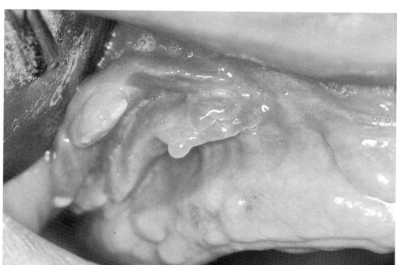

Fig. **75**. Epulis fissuratum.

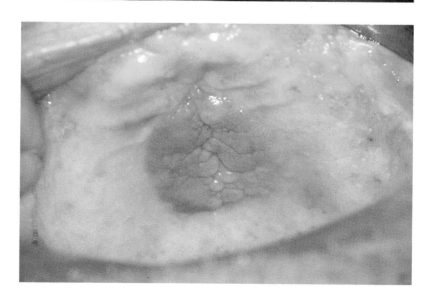

Fig. **76**. Papillary hyperplasia of the palate.

Hyperplasia due to Negative Pressure

In patients wearing dentures, a heart-shaped or round area of mucosal hyperplasia may appear on the hard palate. The mucosa may be slightly elevated and appears red with a smooth or papillary surface (Fig. **77**). This lesion occurs if a relief chamber exists at the center of the basal plate of the denture. The oral mucosal hyperplasia occurs in response to the negative pressure that develops.

Treatment. No treatment is necessary.

Atrophy of the Maxillary Alveolar Ridge

Atrophy of the maxillary alveolar ridge may be the result of excessive occlusal trauma due to a poor fitting denture. It occurs more frequently in women in the anterior maxilla.

The alveolus becomes flabby and red (Fig. **78**).
Epulis fissuratum may coexist.

Treatment. Surgical correction is recommended.

Foreign Body Reaction

Foreign bodies lodged in the oral soft tissues may cause reactive lesions.

The most frequent foreign bodies causing such a reaction are sutures, paraffin, silicon salts, bony fragments, amalgam, metallic fragments from shrapnel, car accidents, etc. The lesions may appear as discolorations, small tumorous enlargements of tissue, abscesses, etc. In peacetime, shrapnel-induced lesions are uncommon. Figure **79** shows a black, well-circumscribed, and asymptomatic nodule caused by shrapnel after a land mine explosion during World War II.

The differential diagnosis includes malignant melanoma, pigmented nevi, and hemangiomas.

Laboratory test. The histopathologic examination is diagnostic, showing reactive granulation tissue and the foreign body fragments. Radiographic examination may be also helpful.

Treatment. Surgical excision.

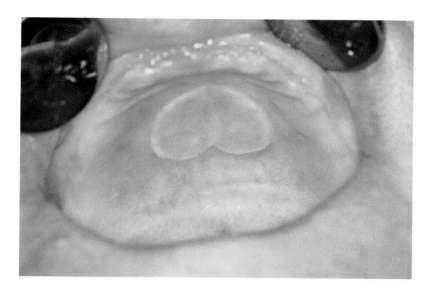

Fig. **77**. Palatal hyperplasia caused by negative pressure.

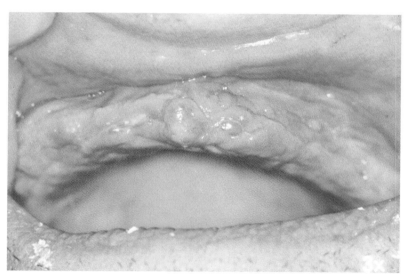

Fig. **78**. Atrophy of the maxillary alveolar ridge.

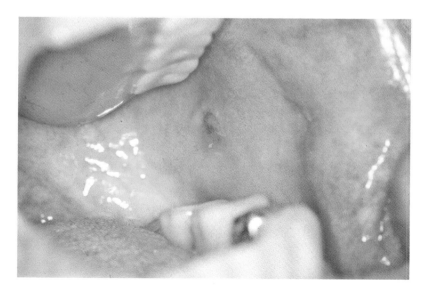

Fig. **79**. Nodule on the buccal mucosa caused by shrapnel after a land mine explosion.

Palatal Necrosis due to Injection

Necrosis of the hard palate may occur after local anesthetic injection. Rapid injection results in local ischemia, which may be followed by necrosis. The hard palate is particularly sensitive to these lesions due to local pressure, because of the firm adherence of mucosa to the bone and the absence of loose connective tissue.

A circular ulcer, a few millimeters in diameter, that heals spontaneously within 2 weeks, is the cardinal manifestation (Fig. **80**).

The differential diagnosis includes necrotizing sialometaplasia and lesions of traumatic origin.

Treatment. Usually, no therapy is necessary. Mouthwashes with oxygen-releasing substrates are recommended.

Eosinophilic Ulcer

Eosinophilic ulcer of the oral mucosa, or eosinophilic granuloma of the oral soft tissues is considered a self-limiting benign lesion unrelated to either facial granuloma or the eosinophilic granuloma of histiocytosis X. The etiology of eosinophilic ulcer remains obscure, although a traumatic background has been suggested. In a series of 25 cases recently reviewed this disease was more frequent in men than women (5.25:1), with a mean age of occurrence of 39 years. The tongue was involved in 74% of the cases and less often the lips, palate, and gingiva. Clinically, the lesions appear as painful ulcers with irregular surface, covered with a whitish-yellow membrane, and raised indurated margins (Figs. **81, 82**).

The sudden onset and pain is a cause of concern for the patient. The ulcer may be single or multiple.

The differential diagnosis includes squamous cell carcinoma, major aphthous ulcers, syphilis, tuberculosis, traumatic ulcer, necrotizing sialometaplasia, Wegener's granulomatosis, lethal midline granuloma, lymphoma, and leukemia.

Laboratory test important to establish the diagnosis is histopathologic examination.

Treatment. Low-dose corticosteroids or surgical excision are helpful. Spontaneous healing after biopsy has occurred occasionally.

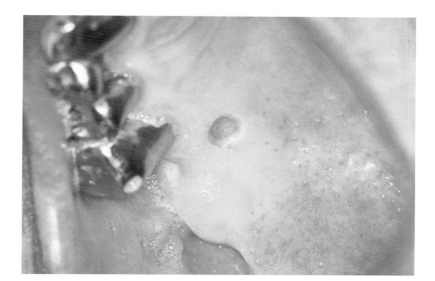

Fig. **80**. Palatal necrosis caused by injection.

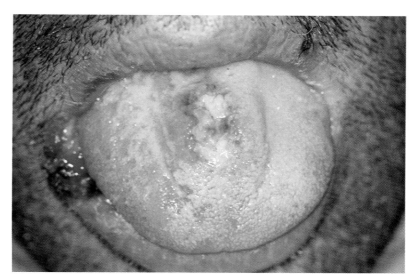

Fig. **81**. Eosinophilic ulcer of the tongue.

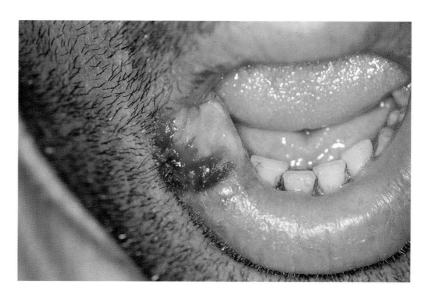

Fig. **82**. Eosinophilic ulcer on the lower lip and the commissure.

5. Oral Lesions due to Chemical Agents

Phenol Burn

Inappropriate or careless use of chemical agents in dental practice may cause oral lesions. Some of these agents may be introduced into the mouth by the patient. The severity of the lesion depends on the type of chemical agent utilized and the concentration and duration of contact of the noxious agent with the tissues. Phenol is used in dentistry as an antiseptic or for local cautery. It is an extremely caustic chemical agent and careless application may cause tissue necrosis. Clinically, there is a whitish surface that later desquamates, exposing a painful erosion or ulcer that heals slowly (Fig. **83**).

The history and clinical appearance of the lesion is diagnostic.

Trichloroacetic Acid Burn

Trichloroacetic acid burns were frequent in the past because this agent was used for cautery of the gingiva. It is an extremely caustic agent, and improper use may result in serious chemical burns. Clinically, there is a white surface due to tissue necrosis (Fig. **84**). Underneath, there is inflammation and erosion or ulceration. The lesion usually heals spontaneously after 1 to 2 weeks.

The differential diagnosis includes chemical burns due to other agents, physical trauma, other necrotic white lesions, and candidosis.

Eugenol Burn

Eugenol is used as an antiseptic and local pulp anesthetic in dentistry. The noxious potential of the drug is limited but may on occasion cause a mucosal burn. Eugenol burns appear as a white-brownish surface with an underlying erosion (Fig. **85**). The lesion heals spontaneously within a week.

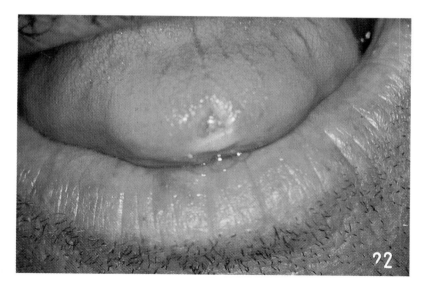

Fig. **83**. Phenol burn.

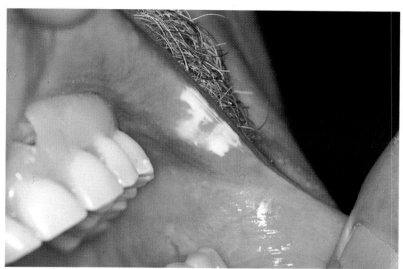

Fig. **84**. Trichloroacetic acid burn.

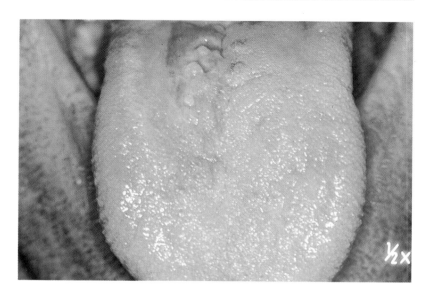

Fig. **85**. Eugenol burn.

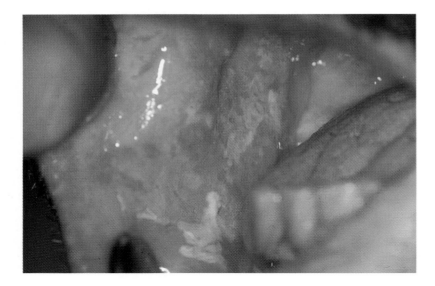

Fig. **86**. Aspirin burn.

Aspirin Burn

Aspirin is sometimes used by patients to relieve
dental pain. Some patients apply aspirin tablets
repeatedly and directly on the painful tooth or on
adjacent tissues. In these cases the drug dissolves
locally causing necrosis of the tissues. The mucosa
is whitish and wrinkled (Fig. **86**). Later, the
necrotic epithelium desquamates exposing an
underlying painful erosion, which heals within a
week.

Iodine Burn

Mild burns may occur after repeated application
of concentrated alcoholic iodine solutions. The
affected mucosa is whitish or red and has a rough
surface (Fig. **87**). The lesion heals spontaneously
within 2 to 4 days.

Alcohol Burn

Concentrated alcohol in the form of absolute
alcohol, or spirits with high alcohol content, is
used on occasion by patients as a local anesthetic
for dental pain. With repeated application, a mild
burn may result. The affected mucosa is whitish,
wrinkled and tender (Fig. **88**). The lesion heals
within 2 to 4 days.

Acrylic Resin Burn

Autopolymerizing acrylic resins are used in dentistry for the construction of temporary prostheses
and may cause local burns either due to heat
evolving during polymerization or to monomer
excess. The mucosa is red with or without erosions
(Fig. **89**).

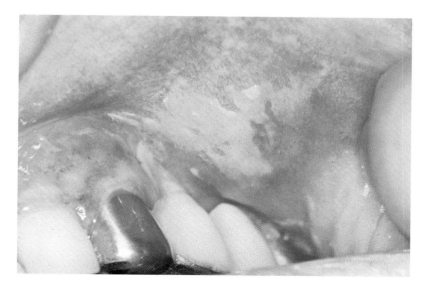

Fig. **87**. Iodine burn.

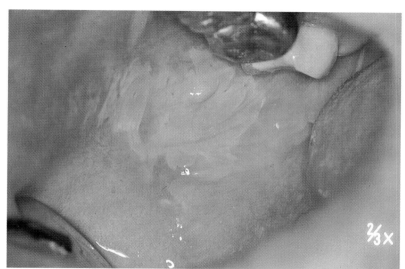

Fig. **88**. Alcohol burn.

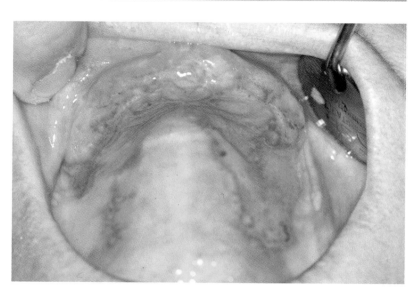

Fig. **89**. Acrylic resin burn.

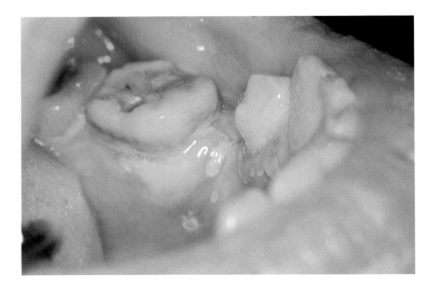

Fig. **90**. Sodium perborate burn.

Sodium Perborate Burn

Sodium perborate has been used as an antiseptic and hemostatic mouthwash. With repeated use, however, it can cause a burn on the oral mucosa that is manifested as an erythematous and edematous area or rarely as a superficial erosion that heals spontaneously (Fig. **90**).

Silver Nitrate Burn

Silver nitrate was used in the past by dentists and otolaryngologists as a cavity sterilizing agent or for cautery of various oral lesions. At the site of application, it creates a painful burn with a whitish or brown surface and erosion (Fig. **91**). Silver nitrate has no place in modern practice.

Sodium Hypochlorite Burn

Sodium hypochlorite is used in endodontics for mechanical irrigation of root canals and as a mild antiseptic. In contact with the oral mucosa, it may cause a mild burn (Fig. **92**). The affected mucosa is red and painful, with superficial erosions that heal spontaneously within 4 to 6 days.

Paraformaldehyde Burn

Paraformaldehyde was used in the past for pulp mummification. It is an extremely caustic chemical agent and in contact with the oral mucosa it may cause severe necrosis of oral tissues (Fig. **93**). The lesions heal within 1 to 2 weeks. Paraformaldehyde has no place in modern endodontic practice.

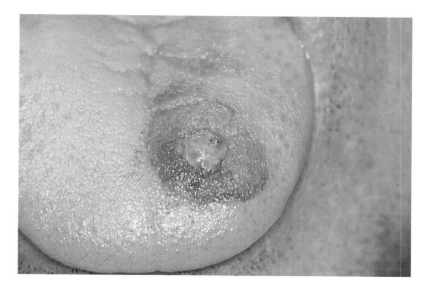

Fig. **91**. Silver nitrate burn.

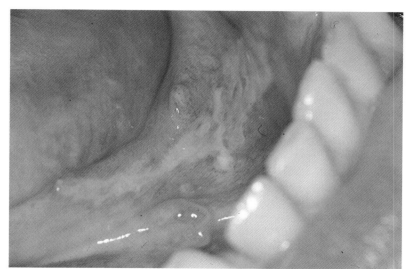

Fig. **92**. Sodium hypochlorite burn.

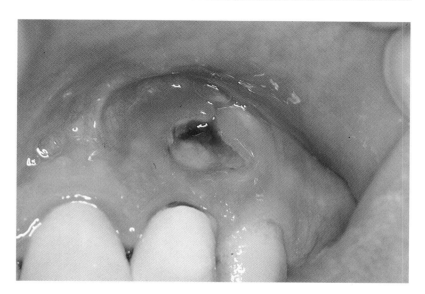

Fig. **93**. Paraformaldehyde burn.

6. Oral Lesions due to Heat

Nicotinic Stomatitis

Nicotinic stomatitis, or smoker's palate, occurs almost exclusively in heavy pipe smokers and only rarely in cigarette or cigar smokers. Thermal and chemical agents acting locally are responsible for the occurrence of this condition. Clinically, nicotinic stomatitis is manifested with redness on the palate, which later assumes a grayish-white and multinodular appearance due to keratinization of the epithelium.

A characteristic finding is the appearance of multiple red dots, 1 to 5 mm in diameter, which represent the dilated and inflamed orifices of minor salivary gland ducts. In heavy smokers there are fissures, furrows, and elevations forming an irregular wrinkled surface (Figs. **94, 95**).

Nicotinic stomatitis is not a precancerous lesion and has a good prognosis. However, it should not be confused with lesions associated with reversed smoking, which have serious consequences and high risk of malignant transformation.

Laboratory test. Histopathologic examination may show a characteristic pattern.

Treatment. Cessation of smoking.

Palatal Erosions due to Smoking

In heavy smokers consuming more than 60 cigarettes a day, palatal painful erosions may occur in addition to nicotinic stomatitis (Fig. **96**). The erosions are due to the elevated temperature in the oral cavity for a long time. Thickening of the epithelium and white lesions may also occur (Fig. **97**).

The differential diagnosis includes traumatic erosions, chemical burns, erythroplakia, and rarely other specific erosions.

Treatment. Cessation of smoking and biopsy to rule out epithelial dysplasia or carcinoma.

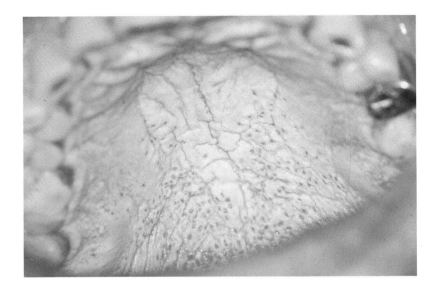

Fig. **94**. Nicotinic stomatitis.

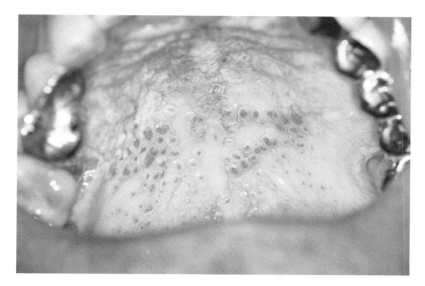

Fig. **95**. Nicotinic stomatitis.

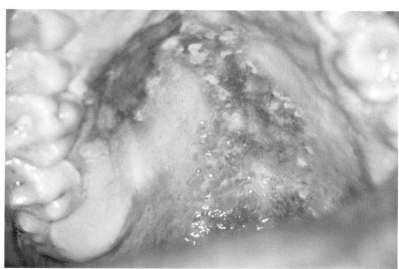

Fig. **96**. Palatal erosions caused by smoking.

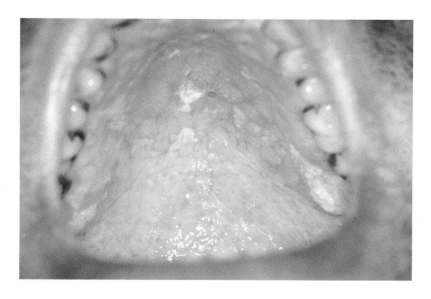

Fig. **97**. Erythema and white lesions on the palate caused by smoking.

Cigarette Smoker's Lip Lesion

Cigarette smoker's lip lesion appears commonly in smokers of nonfiltered cigarettes who hold them between the lips for a long time until short cigarette butts remain. The lesions characteristically appear on the mucosal surface of the lower and upper lips. It is a common finding in psychiatric patients.

The lip lesions correspond to the site at which the cigarette is held and are characterized by flat or slightly elevated whitish areas with red striations (Fig. **98**).

Treatment. Cessation or reduction of smoking.

Thermal Burn

Thermal burns of the oral mucosa are rare. However, very hot foods (such as pizzas, melted cheese), liquid, or hot metal objects may produce mild or severe thermal burns. The palate, lips, floor of the mouth, and tongue are most frequently affected. Clinically, the oral mucosa is painful, red, and may undergo desquamation, leaving small or extensive erosions (Fig. **99**). Vesicles may also appear. The lesions heal in about 1 week. The history is very important in order to make the correct diagnosis. The patient usually remembers the incident that caused the burn.

The differential diagnosis includes chemical burns, traumatic ulcers, aphthous ulcers, herpes simplex, stomatitis medicamentosa, and fellatio.

Treatment. Supportive treatment is recommended.

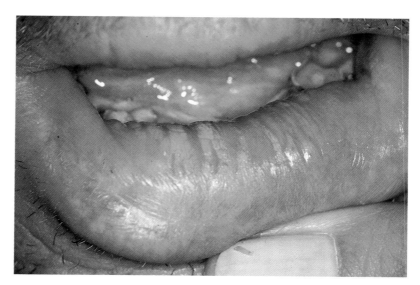

Fig. **98**. Cigarette smoker's lip lesions.

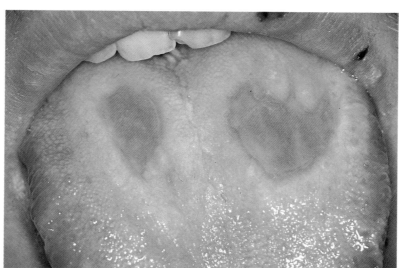

Fig. **99**. Erosions on the dorsum of the tongue caused by very hot food.

7. Oral Lesions due to Drugs

Gold-Induced Stomatitis

Gold compounds are used selectively in patients with rheumatoid disorders. Gold is stored in the tissues and is excreted slowly through the kidneys. Measurable amounts can be detected in the urine 8 to 10 months after cessation of the drug. Gold toxicity may be manifested with fever, headache, proteinuria, skin rashes, oral lesions, thrombocytopenia, agranulocytosis, or aplastic anemia. The oral mucosa is red, with painful erosions covered with a yellowish membrane (Fig. **100**). There is an intense burning sensation and increased salivation. The diagnosis is based on the history and clinical features.

The differential diagnosis includes stomatitis medicamentosa, erythema multiforme, pemphigus vulgaris, cicatricial pemphigoid, bullous pemphigoid, and erosive lichen planus.

Treatment. Cessation of gold therapy. Antihistamines and low-dose steroids may be helpful.

Antibiotic-Induced Stomatitis

Systemic long-term administration of broad-spectrum antibiotics, such as tetracycline, may cause a form of stomatitis. Clinically, it is characterized by a nonspecific diffuse erythema of the oral mucosa. The tongue is extremely red and painful, with desquamation of the filiform papillae (Fig. **101**). Hairy tongue and candidosis may also occur as a result of changes in the oral microbial flora.

The differential diagnosis includes stomatitis medicamentosa, erythema multiforme, pellagra, and ariboflavinosis.

Treatment. Interruption or change of antibiotics and B-complex vitamins are recommended. In the case of candidosis nystatin is indicated.

Stomatitis Medicamentosa

Systemic administration of medications may induce hypersensitivity reactions in the oral mucosa characterized as stomatitis medicamentosa, or pharmaceutical stomatitis.

A plethora of drugs may cause stomatitis medicamentosa, including antipyretics, sulfonamides, antibiotics, and barbiturates. Clinically, the condition is characterized by diffuse erythema of the oral mucosa, purpuric patches, vesicles or bullae, painful erosions, ulcers, etc. (Fig. **102**). Any area of the mouth may be involved. The lesions appear during or shortly after administration of a drug and may recur.

The differential diagnosis includes erythema multiforme, pemphigus, bullous pemphigoid, cicatricial pemphigoid, erosive and bullous lichen planus, etc.

Treatment. Cessation of the drug. Antihistamines or steroids in low doses.

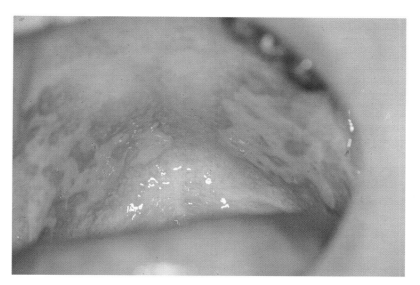

Fig. **100**. Gold-induced stomatitis, erosions on the palate.

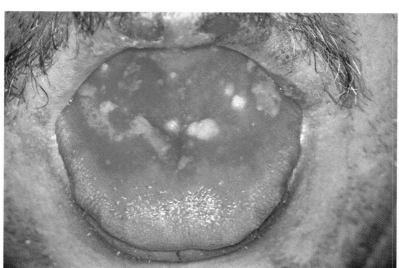

Fig. **101**. Antibiotic-induced stomatitis, diffuse erythema and desquamation of the filiform papillae of the tongue.

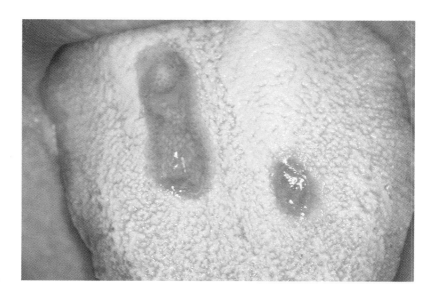

Fig. **102**. Stomatitis medicamentosa, erosions on the dorsum of the tongue.

Ulcerations due to Methotrexate

Methotrexate is a folic acid antimetabolite that is used in the treatment of leukemias, solid cancers, psoriasis, etc. Side effects occur by inhibiting the formation of nucleic acid in both malignant and normal cells. The most common side effects are alopecia, liver and gastrointestinal disorders, etc. Oral mucosal lesions are frequent and are characterized by redness and painful erosions or ulcers (Fig. **103**). They commonly involve the tongue, lips, and buccal mucosa, although they may occur anywhere in the oral cavity.

These lesions appear 2 to 3 weeks after initiation of treatment and constitute an indication for cessation of drug or lowering of the dose.

The differential diagnosis includes traumatic ulcer, thermal and chemical burn, stomatitis medicamentosa.

Treatment. Folic acid replacement and changing the drug, if possible.

Ulceration due to Azathioprine

Azathioprine is an antimetabolite widely used as an immunosuppressive drug. Alopecia, gastrointestinal disorders, and bone marrow toxicity are the most common side effects. Rarely, limited erosions or ulcers of the oral mucosa may develop after long-term and high-dose administration (Fig. **104**).

Treatment. Lowering the dose of the drug, and B-complex vitamin administration.

Penicillamine-Induced Oral Lesions

D-penicillamine, a heavy metal chelator used in the treatment of hepatolenticular degeneration (Wilson's disease) and other diseases (rheumatoid arthritis, primary biliary cirrhosis, scleroderma, cystinuria, and heavy metal intoxication), may be associated with mucocutaneous and noncutaneous side effects. The noncutaneous side effects include hematologic, pulmonary, gastrointestinal, renal, autoimmune, and allergic disorders. The most common cutaneous manifestations are autoimmune disorders (pemphigus group, cicatricial pemphigoid, lupus erythematosus), acute sensitivity reaction, interference with collagen and elastin, etc. The most common oral manifestation is penicillamine-induced pemphigus, which is characterized by vesiculobullous lesions and erosions of the oral mucosa, clinically, histopathologically, and immunologically identical to those seen in classic pemphigus. Commonly, involvement of the oral mucosa may be the first sign of the disease and rarely the only manifestation (Fig. **105**). Penicillamine-induced pemphigus usually appears within 6 to 12 months after initiation of the drug and may resolve within several weeks after withdrawal of the drug. Cicatricial pemphigoid lesions, aphthous stomatitis, and taste loss are also oral complications of the drug. Pemphigus and cicatricial pemphigoid lesions are frequently seen in penicillamine-treated patients with rheumatoid arthritis.

The differential diagnosis of oral lesions includes classic pemphigus, cicatricial pemphigoid, bullous pemphigoid, erythema multiforme, and stomatitis medicamentosa.

Treatment is withdrawal of penicillamine and systemic steroids.

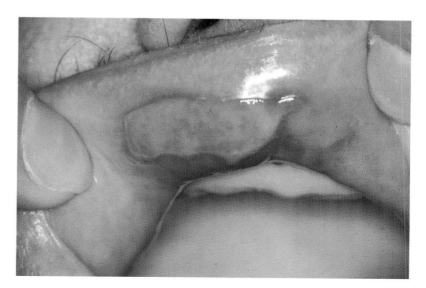

Fig. **103**. Ulcer on the upper lip caused by methotrexate.

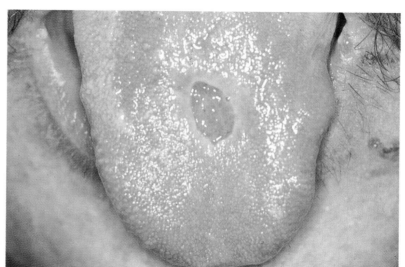

Fig. **104**. Ulcer on the tongue caused by azathioprine.

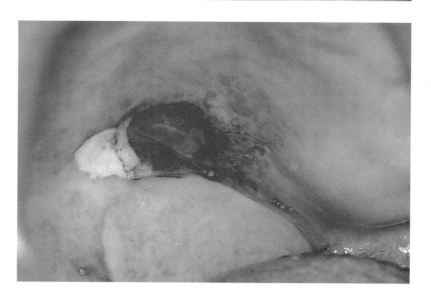

Fig. **105**. Penicillamine-induced oral pemphigus, erosion on the palate.

Fibrous Gingival Hyperplasia due to Phenytoin

Phenytoin is an antiepileptic agent widely used in patients with generalized seizures.

A common side effect is fibrous gingival hyperplasia, which occurs in 30 to 60% of the patients taking the drug. Although the exact mechanism of gingival hyperplasia is not clear, the appearance and degree of the hyperplasia depend on the daily dose, the duration of therapy, the state of oral hygiene, and other local and systemic factors. The hyperplasia usually begins in the interdental papillae and gradually involves the marginal and attached gingiva. With gradual progression, the gingiva may cover the crowns of the teeth entirely.

The gingivae are firm, lobulated, slightly red, and painless, with little or no tendency to bleed (Fig. 106). Usually, the enlargement of the gingiva is generalized. Rarely, hyperplasia may occur in edentulous patients.

The differential diagnosis includes cyclosporine-induced hyperplasia, idiopathic fibromatosis of the gingiva, and gingival hypertrophy due to mouth breathing or leukemia.

Treatment. Careful oral hygiene, surgical excision. Discontinuation of the drug or change to another antiepileptic agent may result in regression of the hyperplasia.

Fibrous Gingival Hyperplasia due to Cyclosporine

Cyclosporine is a powerful immunosuppressive drug used to prevent organ transplant rejection and to treat lupus erythematosus and many other autoimmune diseases. Several side effects of cyclosporine have been reported, such as hepatotoxicity, nephrotoxicity, hirsutism, mild tremor, and predisposition to cancers. Gingival hyperplasia is a common side effect occurring in about 70% of the patients receiving cyclosporine therapy. Cyclosporine-induced gingival hyperplasia is related to the time of therapy, the serum concentration of the drug, and the presence of dental plaque. It is more common in children and adolescents than adults, and the degree of gingival enlargement may vary from mild or moderate to severe. Clinically, the gingiva is enlarged, firm with focal lobulation, and little inflammation (Fig. 107).

The differential diagnosis includes fibrous gingival hyperplasia due to phenytoin, gingival fibromatosis, gingivitis, periodontitis, and leukemia.

Treatment. Gingivectomy. The lesions are usually reversible after cessation of the drug.

Angioneurotic Edema

Angioneurotic edema is a common allergic reaction that may be acquired or inherited. The inherited form is associated with C1 esterase inhibitor deficiency and is inherited as an autosomal dominant trait. In addition to sudden facial edema, edema of the larynx and tongue, which involves the gastrointestinal tract, with abdominal pain, nausea, vomiting, and diarrhea, also occur. The acquired form is far more frequent and may be due to food allergy, pharmaceuticals, local anesthetics, infections, and emotional stress. These factors may act either directly on mast cells or through an immunoglobulin E-mediated allergic reaction to cause release of inflammatory mediators, such as histamine, kinins, and leukotrienes. The result is capillary leakage and submucosal or subcutaneous edema.

Angioneurotic edema of either type has a sudden onset, lasts usually for 24 to 48 hours, and may recur at variable time intervals. Clinically, it is characterized by painless, usually nonpruritic and smooth swelling involving the lips (Fig. 108), tongue, soft palate, face, hands, feet, or any other area. Edema of the glottis represents a severe complication that may result in death.

The differential diagnosis should include trauma, surgical emphysema, cellulitis, cheilitis granulomatosa, Melkersson-Rosenthal syndrome, and cheilitis glandularis.

Treatment. Antihistamines, systemic steroids, and in acute severe cases epinephrine subcutaneously.

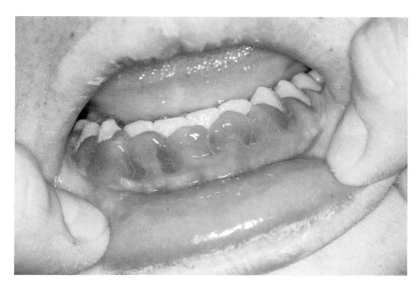

Fig. **106**. Fibrous gingival hyperplasia caused by phenytoin.

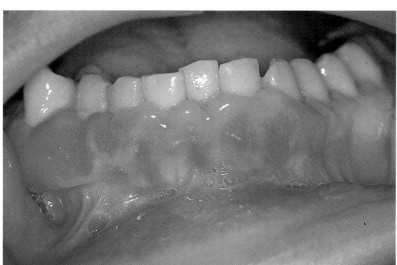

Fig. **107**. Gingival hyperplasia caused by cyclosporine.

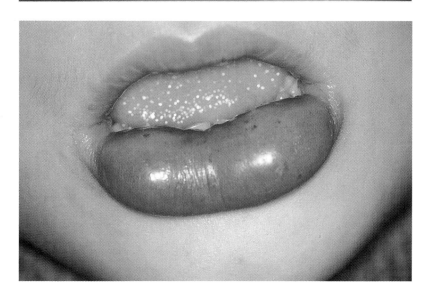

Fig. **108**. Angioneurotic edema, swelling of the lower lip.

Pigmentation due to Antimalarials

Chloroquine and other antimalarials are used in the treatment of malaria and occasionally in patients with rheumatoid arthritis and lupus erythamatosus. Long-term use may cause brown or black irregular pigmentation on the soft palate or other areas of the oral cavity (Fig. **109**). These discolorations must be differentiated from Addison's disease and usually remit with interruption of the drug.

Cheilitis due to Retinoids

During the last decade, synthetic retinoids (13-cis-retinoic acid and the aromatic analogue of retinoic acid, etretinate) have been introduced as new agents in the modern therapy of skin diseases. They are extremely effective drugs in various dis-orders of keratinization. In addition, they have anti-inflammatory and immunomodulatory effects. Synthetic retinoids have recently been used in the treatment of psoriasis, acne vulgaris, ichthyosis, lichen planus, parapsoriasis en plaques, mycosis fungoides, Darier's disease, and other keratotic genodermatoses.

Several side effects may appear during retinoid administration. The most common are dryness with scaling of the lips and dryness of the oral mucosa (Fig. **110**). Hair loss, palmoplantar scaling, thinning of the skin, pruritus, epistaxis, paronychia, and vomiting may also occur. No severe complications have been observed after retinoid administration in therapeutic dosages. However, pregnancy must be avoided during and 1 year after treatment because of the teratogenic and embryotoxic action of these drugs.

Treatment. Cheilitis and dryness of the mouth remit after discontinuing the drugs.

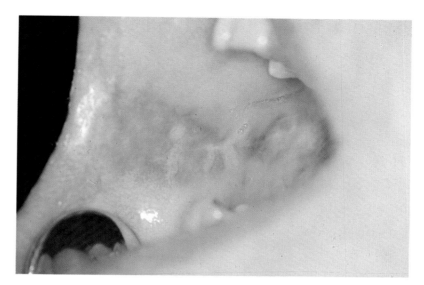

Fig. **109**. Pigmentation of the buccal mucosa caused by chloroquine.

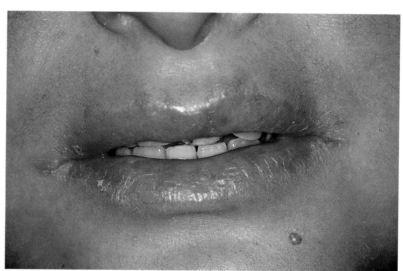

Fig. **110**. Cheilitis caused by systemic administration of the aromatic retinoid etretinate.

8. Metal and Other Deposits

Amalgam Tattoo

Amalgam deposition develops either as a result of continuous contact between an amalgam filling and the gingiva or from embedding of amalgam fragments in the oral tissues during dental filling or surgical operations. In addition, during tooth extraction, fragments of amalgam restorations are broken off and may be embedded in the adjacent soft tissues. Amalgam tattoo appears as a well-defined flat area with a bluish-black or brownish discoloration of varying size (Fig. 111). Amalgam deposits usually occur in the gingiva, the alveolar mucosa, and the buccal mucosa.

The differential diagnosis includes pigmented nevi, malignant melanoma, normal pigmentation, and hematoma.

Laboratory test. Histopathologic examination and radiographs are necessary on occasion to differentiate amalgam tattoo from other lesions of the oral mucosa with dark discoloration.

Treatment. No treatment is required.

Bismuth Deposition

Bismuth compounds were formely used in the treatment of syphilis. However, in recent years antibiotics have replaced these compounds in the treatment of syphilis. Oral discolorations due to bismuth are now rarely encountered except in patients who have been treated for syphilis in the preantibiotic era and have poor oral hygiene. Clinically, bismuth deposition forms a characteristic bluish line along the marginal gingiva or black spots within the gingival papillae (Fig. 112). Less frequently, bismuth may be deposited in other areas of the oral mucosa, mainly the periphery of ulcers or in areas of inflammation.

The differential diagnosis includes normal pigmentation, silver deposition, amalgam tattoo, and Addison's disease.

Treatment. No treatment is required.

Materia Alba of the Attached Gingiva

Materia alba is the result of accumulation of bacteria, dead epithelial cells, and food debris. It is usually found at the dentogingival margins of persons with poor oral hygiene. However, materia alba presenting as a white plaque along the vestibular surface of the gingiva and the alveolar mucosa may be seen in patients who are unable to brush their teeth because of painful oral diseases (Fig. 113). The white plaque is soft and easily detatched after slight pressure, leaving a red surface.

The differential diagnosis should include leukoplakia and candidosis.

Treatment is good oral hygiene.

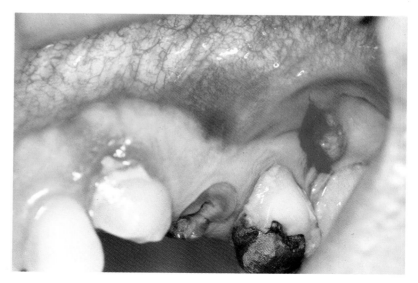

Fig. **111**. Amalgam tattoo.

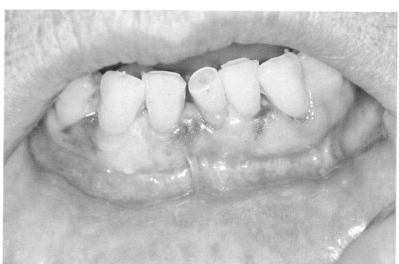

Fig. **112**. Bismuth deposition within the gingival papillae.

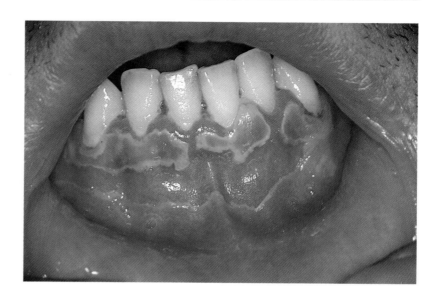

Fig. **113**. White plaques on the attached gingiva and the alveolar mucosa caused by materia alba accumulation.

9. Radiation-Induced Injuries

Radiation therapy has a prominent place in the treatment of oral and other head and neck cancers. The most common form of radiation used is ionizing radiation, delivered by an external source, or radioactive implants (gold, iridium, etc.).

Ionizing radiation, in addition to its therapeutic effect, can also affect normal tissues. The oral mucosal side effects after radiation are mainly dependent on the dose and the duration of treatment. These radiation-induced mucosal reactions may be classified as early and late. Early reactions appear at the end of the first week of therapy and consist of erythema and edema of the oral mucosa. During the second week, erosions and ulcers may appear, which are covered by a whitish-yellow exudate (Figs. **114, 115**). Subjective complaints include malaise, xerostomia, loss of taste, burning, and pain during mastication, speech, and swallowing. The lesions persist during the treatment period and for several weeks thereafter. If the salivary glands are irradiated, xerostomia is one of the earliest and most common findings. Spontaneous remission of oral lesions may occur gradually after termination of the radiation treatment. However, secondary infection may delay recovery. Late manifestations are usually irreversible and result in extremely sensitive atrophic oral mucosa. The teeth, in the absence of salivary protection, rapidly develop caries and finally are destroyed (Fig. **116**). Osteoradionecrosis is a serious complication and occurs in cases of high-dose radiation, especially if inadequate measures are taken to reduce the radiation dosage delivered to the bones. It is manifested as painful osteomyelitis with bone necrosis and sequestration and, rarely, formation of extraoral fistulas. The mandible is more frequently affected than the maxilla. The risk of this complication is increased particularly if teeth within the radiation field are extracted after irradiation.

Diagnosis of oral lesions due to radiation depends on the medical history and the clinical features.

Treatment should include preventive measures, cessation of the radiation therapy, analgesics, topical steroids, anti-inflammatory agents, B-complex vitamins, and antibiotics in case of oral mucosa and bone infections.

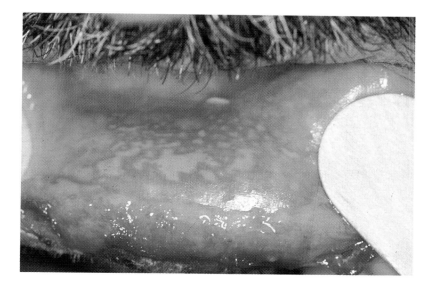

Fig. **114**. Erythema and erosions on the lower lip caused by ionizing radiation.

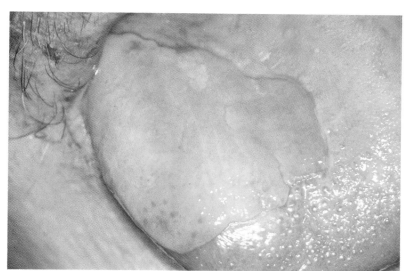

Fig. **115**. Erosion on the tongue caused by radioactive iridium.

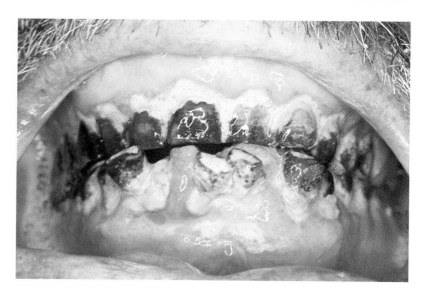

Fig. **116**. Dental and gingival lesions caused by ionizing radiation.

10. Allergy to Chemical Agents Applied Locally

Allergic Stomatitis due to Acrylic Resin

True allergy of the oral mucosa to denture base material is very rare. The residual acrylic monomer (methyl methacrylate), however, is believed to be responsible for allergic reactions of the oral mucosa in susceptible persons. Alternatively, traces of other allergenic substances absorbed within the denture base may be the cause of the allergic reactions.

Allergic acrylic stomatitis is characterized by diffuse erythema, edema, and occasionally small vesicles and erosions, especially in areas of contact with the dentures (Figs. **117, 118**). The patient complains of intense burning of the mouth and this reaction may extend to areas of the oral mucosa that are not in direct contact with the dentures. Removal of the dentures usually results in complete resolution. The skin patch test is usually positive.

The differential diagnosis includes denture stomatitis and reactions to other allergens.

Treatment consists of oral antihistamines and construction of new dentures with fully polymerized monomer.

Allergic Stomatitis due to Eugenol

Eugenol has many uses in dentistry as an antiseptic, filling material, and periodontal pack. In sensitized patients it may cause generalized allergic reactions after direct contact with the oral mucosa.

In localized reactions there is redness, edema, and erosions that are covered with whitish pseudomembranes (Fig. **119**). Subjectively, there is intense pain. The skin patch test is usually positive.

Treatment consists of removal of the eugenol and the use of antihistamines.

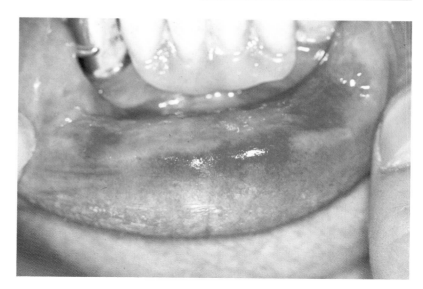

Fig. **117**. Allergic stomatitis caused by acrylic resin.

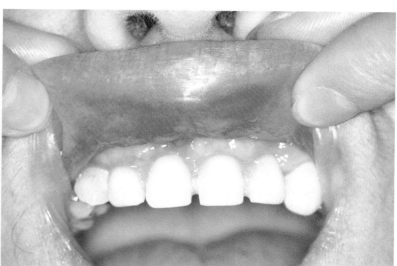

Fig. **118**. Allergic stomatitis caused by acrylic resin.

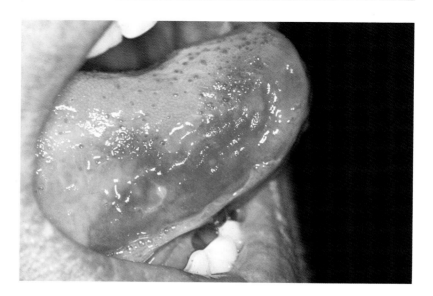

Fig. **119**. Allergic stomatitis caused by eugenol.

11. Periodontal Diseases

Gingivitis

Gingivitis is an inflammatory disease of the gingiva caused by dental microbial plaque. Factors that contribute to the accumulation of plaque are poor oral hygiene, faulty restorations, tooth malposition, calculus, food impaction, mouth breathing, etc. In addition, several systemic disorders, such as endocrine diseases, immune deficiencies, nutritional disturbances, and drugs, are known to be modifying factors of host response to the microbial activity of plaque. The severity of gingivitis is related to local factors and the host resistance. Clinically, the gingiva appear red and swollen, with decreased and finally loss of normal stippling. An early and common feature is gingival bleeding, even after mild local stimulation. Inflammation is mainly located at the marginal gingiva and the interdental papillae without development of periodontal pockets (Fig. **120**). However, if gingival hyperplasia is severe, pseudopockets may be formed. Gingivitis is frequently chronic, although occasionally acute or subacute forms may occur. If chronic gingivitis is not treated, it frequently evolves into periodontitis.

Treatment. Good oral hygiene, complete removal of calculus from the teeth, and repair of faulty restorations are indicated.

Periodontitis

Periodontitis is a chronic inflammatory disease that involves all periodontal tissues (gingiva, periodontal ligament, cementum, alveolar bone) and usually follows chronic gingivitis. Local factors also contribute to the development of periodontitis, but the most important factor is host resistance to local infection. Recently, an aggressive form of periodontitis has been recorded in patients with acquired immune deficiency syndrome. The cardinal clinical features of periodontitis are periodontal pocket formation and alveolar bone loss. Other findings include gingival swelling, redness and bleeding, gingival hyperplasia or recession, pyorrhea, varying degree of tooth mobility, and migration (Fig. **121**).

Laboratory test. Radiographic examination confirms the diagnosis.

Treatment. The treatment consists of an effective plaque control regimen followed by scaling and root planing, surgical procedures, and, in certain cases, systemic antibiotics.

Juvenile Periodontitis

Juvenile periodontitis is an inflammatory gingival disease that occurs in otherwise healthy children and young adults. Although the exact cause remains obscure, recent evidence suggests that infection by local specific microorganisms and host response play important roles in the pathogenesis of the disease.

Based on clinical, radiographic, microbiologic, and immunologic criteria, juvenile periodontitis is classified into two forms: localized juvenile periodontitis, which clinically is characterized by severe periodontal pocket formation and alveolar bone loss with mild or moderate inflammation localized mainly in the periodontal tissues of the permanent incisors and first molars, and generalized juvenile periodontitis, which is clinically characterized by generalized periodontal pockets and alveolar bone loss that involves almost all teeth along with gingival inflammation (Fig. **122**).

The differential diagnosis includes juvenile periodontitis associated with several systemic diseases, such as Papillon-Lefèvre syndrome, hypophosphatasia, acatalasemia, histiocytosis X, cyclic neutropenia, agranulocytosis, juvenile diabetes mellitus, Crohn's disease, and Ehlers-Danlos syndrome.

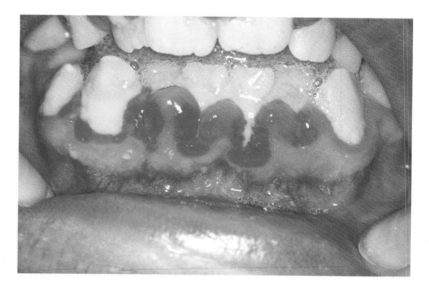

Fig. **120**. Gingivitis.

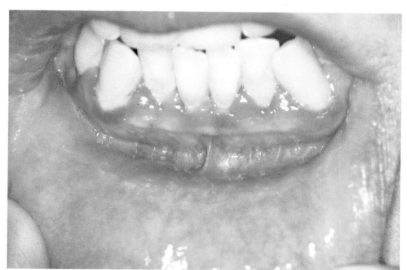

Fig. **121**. Periodontitis.

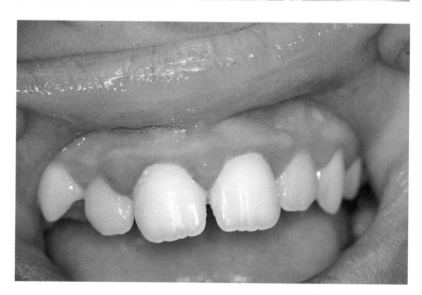

Fig. **122**. Generalized juvenile periodontitis.

Laboratory tests to establish the diagnosis are radiographs, bacterial cultures, and immune studies.

Treatment. The treatment consists of plaque control followed by scaling and root planing, surgical procedures, and systemic antibiotics.

Periodontal Abscess

Periodontal abscess is formed by localized pus accumulation in a preexisting periodontal pocket. When the depth of the periodontal pocket exceeds 5 to 8 mm, the edematous gingival tissues around the cervix of the tooth may approximate the tooth tightly and cause complete obstruction of the opening of the pocket so that a periodontal abscess is formed. Clinically, it appears as a painful soft, red gingival enlargement (Fig. **123**). On pressure, pus exudes from the cervical area of the tooth. The teeth involved are tender to percussion and occasionally mobile. When substantial pus accumulation occurs, it diffuses into the surrounding tissues, resulting in cellulitis. Fever, malaise, and mild lymphadenopathy may be present.

The differential diagnosis includes dental abscess, gingival cyst of adults, palatine papilla cyst, nasolabial cyst, and actinomycosis.

Laboratory test. Radiographic examination may be helpful.

Treatment. Antibiotics during the acute phase and periodontal treatment.

Periodontal Fistula

Periodontal fistula forms when pus bores through the gingival tissues and drains an underlying periodontal abscess. Clinically, the orifice of the fistula appears red, with granulomatous tissue formation (Fig. **124**). On pressure, the orifice will release pus. The pulp of the neighboring teeth is vital.

The differential diagnosis includes periapical abscess and fistula, osteomyelitis, actinomycosis, and tuberculosis.

Treatment consists of surgical procedures, scaling, and root planing.

Gingivitis and Mouth Breathing

Habitual mouth breathing favors the development of gingivitis with some special clinical features. This form of gingivitis affects the vestibular portion of the maxillary anterior gingiva in young persons. Clinically, the gingiva appear swollen, red, dry, and shiny, covering part of the crown of the teeth (Fig. **125**).

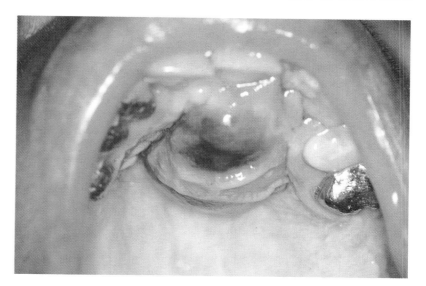

Fig. **123**. Periodontal abscess.

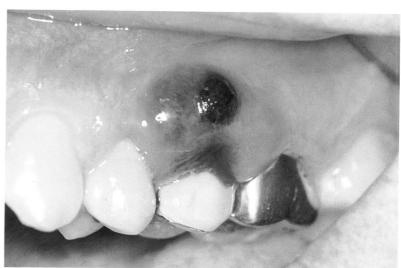

Fig. **124**. Periodontal fistula.

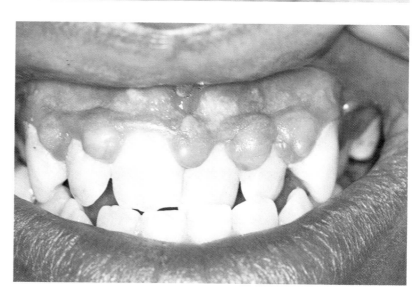

Fig. **125**. Gingivitis caused by mouth breathing.

Plasma Cell Gingivitis

Plasma cell gingivitis is a unique disorder that histopathologically is characterized by a dense plasma cell infiltration of the gingival connective tissue. The disease shows clinical and histopathologic similarities to plasma cell balanitis or Zoon's balanitis. The precise cause remains obscure, although several factors have been incriminated, such as chronic infections, hormonal disorders, allergy, Candida albicans, and hypersensitivity to several components of chewing gum. Plasma cell gingivitis is more common in women between 20 and 50 years of age, and it usually lasts for several months or years. Clinically, both marginal and attached gingiva are bright red and edematous with a faintly stippled surface (Fig. **126**). The gingivitis may be localized or widespread and frequently is accompanied by itching and burning. Similar lesions have been described on the tongue and lips.

The differential diagnosis includes desquamative gingivitis, gingivitis, geographic stomatitis, early leukemic gingival lesions, erythroplasia of Queyrat, candidosis, and psoriasis.

Laboratory test. Histopathologic examination confirms the diagnosis.

Treatment. Specific treatment does not exist. At times, antihistamines and nystatin may be helpful.

Desquamative Gingivitis

Desquamative gingivitis does not represent a specific disease entity, but is a descriptive term used to name a rather nonspecific gingival manifestation of several disease processes. Recent findings suggest that the great majority of cases of desquamative gingivitis represents a manifestation of chronic bullous dermatoses, such as cicatricial pemphigoid, pemphigus vulgaris, bullous pemphigoid, and lichen planus. In a recent study of 453 patients with these disorders we found desquamative gingivitis in 63.6% of the cases with cicatricial pemphigoid, in 25% with lichen planus; in 18.4% with pemphigus vulgaris; and in 3.2% with bullous pemphigoid. Clinically, desquamative gingivitis is characterized by erythema and edema of the marginal and attached gingiva, predominantly labially and buccally (Figs. **127, 128**). A characteristic sign is peeling off of the epithelium or elevation with subsequent formation of a hemorrhagic blister after massage of the gingiva.

The gingival lesions may be either localized or diffuse. Desquamative gingivitis may be the only oral manifestation or may be associated with other oral manifestations of a chronic bullous dermatosis. In the presence of desquamative gingivitis the identification of the underlying disease is based on the following criteria: careful clinical observation of all intraoral and extraoral lesions, histopathologic examination of gingival biopsy specimens, direct immunofluorescence of gingival biopsy specimens, indirect immunofluorescent examination for serum epithelial antibodies, and clinical follow-up of the patient.

The differential diagnosis includes plasma cell gingivitis and chronic mechanical gingival trauma.

Treatment. The therapy of desquamative gingivitis depends on the identification and treatment of the underlying disease.

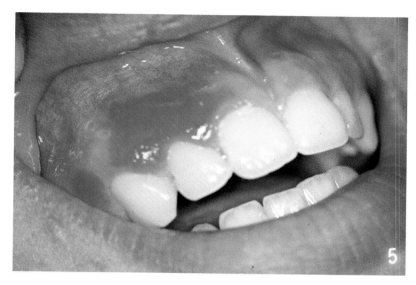

Fig. **126**. Plasma cell gingivitis.

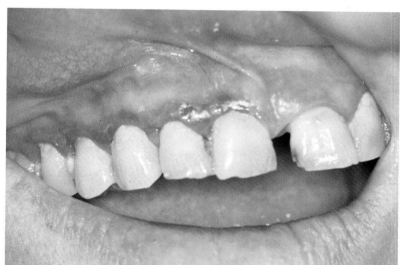

Fig. **127**. Desquamative gingivitis as a manifestation of cicatricial pemphigoid.

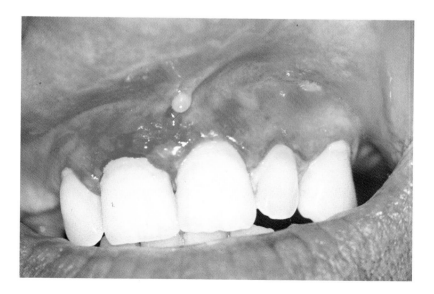

Fig. **128**. Desquamative gingivitis as a manifestation of pemphigus vulgaris.

12. Diseases of the Tongue

Median Rhomboid Glossitis

Median rhomboid glossitis is a congenital abnormality of the tongue that is thought to be due to persistence of the tuberculum impar untill adulthood. The disorder appears on the dorsal surface of the tongue as an area devoid of papillae. However, recently, it has been suggested that chronic Candida albicans infection may play a role in the pathogenesis of median rhomboid glossitis. Clinically, the lesion has a rhomboid or oval shape and is localized along the midline of the dorsum of the tongue immediately anterior to the circumvallate papillae. Two clinical varieties are recognized: a smooth, well-circumscribed red plaque that is devoid of normal papillae, slightly below the level of the surrounding normal mucosa (Fig. **129**), and a raised multinodular, firm, reddish mass with a smooth surface without papillae (Fig. **130**).

Median rhomboid glossitis is usually asymptomatic, although occasionally secondary C. albicans infection may occur with mild inflammation causing subjective symptoms.

The differential diagnosis includes interstitial syphilitic glossitis, candidosis, geographic tongue, thyroglossal duct cyst, lymphangioma, and other neoplasms.

Laboratory test. Histopathologic examination is occasionally indicated to exclude neoplasia.

Treatment is generally not required. In cases of C. albicans infection topical use of nystatin or clotrimazole is helpful.

Geographic Tongue

Geographic tongue, or benign migratory glossitis, is a disorder of unknown cause and pathogenesis, although an inherited pattern has been suggested. The prevalence ranges from 1 to 2%. It appears in all ages and is slightly more common in females. Geographic tongue frequently coexists with fissured tongue. Clinically, the condition is characterized by multiple, usually painless, circinate erythematous patches surrounded by a thin, raised whitish border (Fig. **131**). The lesions vary in size from several millimeters to several centimeters and are due to desquamation of the filiform papillae, whereas the fungiform papillae remain intact and prominent. These lesions persist for a short time in one area and then heal completely and reappear in another area of the tongue.

Geographic tongue is a benign condition persisting for weeks, months, or even years and is usually restricted to the dorsal surface of the tongue. Occasionally, lesions may appear on the ventral surface and the margins. However, similar lesions have also been described in other areas of the oral mucosa (such as lips, buccal mucosa, gingiva) and have been described as geographic stomatitis or migratory stomatitis (Fig. **132**).

The differential diagnosis includes oral lesions of psoriasis and Reiter's syndrome, plasma cell glossitis, mucous patches of secondary syphilis, lichen planus, leukoplakia, candidosis, and allergic reactions.

Treatment is not required. However, patients should be reassured.

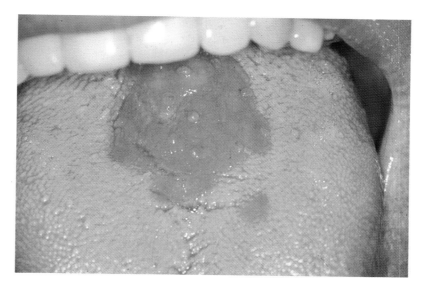

Fig. **129**. Median rhomboid glossitis.

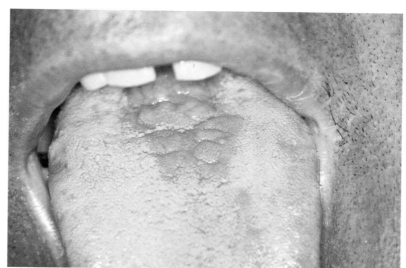

Fig. **130**. Median rhomboid glossitis.

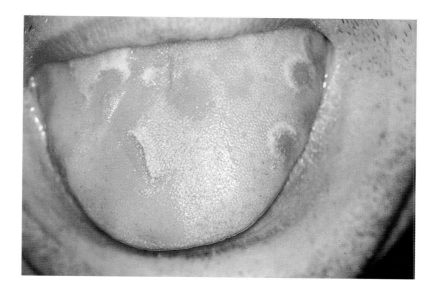

Fig. **131**. Geographic tongue.

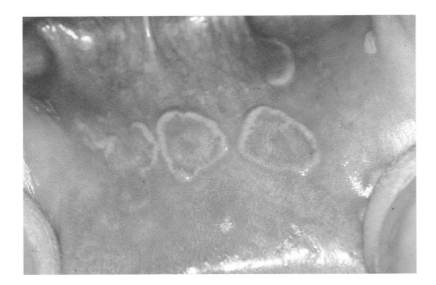

Fig. **132**. Geographic stomatitis, lesions on lower lip mucosa.

Fissured Tongue

Fissured or scrotal tongue is a common developmental malformation of unknown cause and pathogenesis. However, recent evidence supports the concept that fissured and geographic tongues are inherited disorders with a common polygenic mode of transmission. Clinically, fissured tongue is characterized by multiple fissures or grooves on the dorsal surface of the tongue resulting in a scrotal appearance (Fig. **133**). The fissures may vary in depth, size, and number and usually have a symmetrical distribution. The condition is asymptomatic, although food debris, microorganisms, and fungi may be retained in the deeper fissures and may cause mild local irritation. The prevalence ranges from 0.5 to 5%.

Fissured tongue may coexist with geographic tongue and is one of the clinical diagnostic criteria of Melkersson-Rosenthal syndrome. It is also a feature of Down's syndrome.

The differential diagnosis includes tongue appearance in Sjögren's syndrome and interstitial syphilitic glossitis.

Treatment is not required.

Hairy Tongue

Hairy tongue is a relatively common disorder that is due to hypertrophy and elongation of the filliform papillae. The cause is obscure, although several predisposing factors have been incriminated, such as oral antibiotics, oxidizing agents, metronidazole, excessive smoking, radiation, emotional stress, poor oral hygiene, and C. albicans. Clinically, the condition is characterized by hypertrophy and elongation of the filiform papillae of the dorsum of the tongue, which take on a hairy appearance. The color of the filiform papillae may be yellowish-white, brown, or black when pigment-producing bacteria colonize the elongated papillae (Figs. **134, 135**).

The disorder is usually asymptomatic although the excessive length of the papillae may cause an unpleasant feeling in the mouth, such as gagging and discomfort. Although the disorder is benign in nature, it may cause significant distress to the patient for esthetic reasons.

Treatment. In mild cases, brushing of the dorsum of the tongue may promote desquamation and reduce the length of the papillae. Nystatin may be helpful in selected cases, when C. albicans growth is documented. In cases of extreme papillary elongation, topical use of keratolytic agents (such as salicylic acid in alcohol, podophyllin in alcohol, trichloroacetic acid) may be helpful.

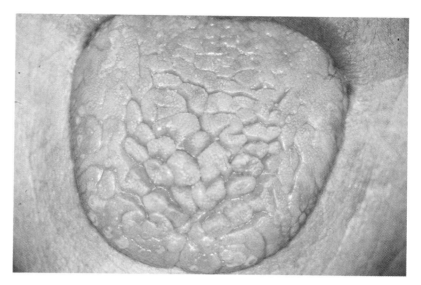

Fig. **133**. Fissured tongue.

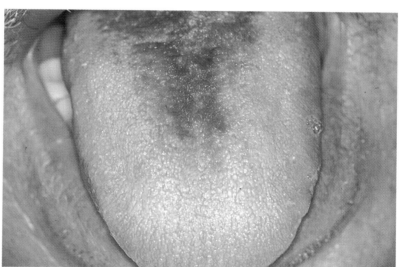

Fig. **134**. Hairy tongue.

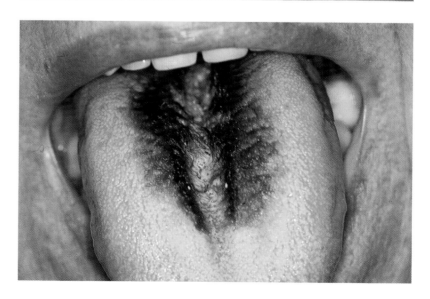

Fig. **135**. Black hairy tongue.

Plasma Cell Glossitis

Plasma cell glossitis is a rare disorder characterized by diffuse or localized erythema of the tongue, which exhibits plasma cell infiltration on histopathologic examination (Fig. **136**).

The cause of the disease is unknown, although several predisposing factors, such as allergic reactions, endocrine disorders, C. albicans, have been incriminated.

Plasma cell glossitis may persist for a prolonged period and may be accompanied by a burning sensation.

Similar lesions may appear on the gingiva, lips, and other areas of the oral mucosa.

The differential diagnosis includes geographic tongue, allergic reactions, and candidosis.

Laboratory test. Histopathologic examination is essential to establish the diagnosis.

Treatment is symptomatic. Antihistamines and nystatin may be helpful.

Glossodynia

Glossodynia, or glossopyrosis is not a specific disease entity but a symptom of burning sensation of the tongue. During the last decades, it has become a very common condition, particularly in women more than 50 years old. In the vast majority glossodynia represents a manifestation of an underlying psychologic problem with no clinically visible changes. Other common causes are candidosis, iron deficiency anemia, pernicious anemia, geographic tongue, lichen planus, xerostomia, diabetes mellitus, hypertension, allergic reaction, etc. In glossodynia of psychologic origin, the tongue is usually normal, although slight erythema and mild elongation of fungiform papillae at the tip of the tongue may occasionally occur (Fig. **137**). The patient complains of a burning sensation or itching, usually at the tip and the lateral borders of the tongue. Similar symptoms may appear at any area of the oral cavity. The condition is, as a rule, associated with cancerophobia, shows remissions and exacerbations, and may persist for years.

Treatment. There is no specific treatment, although various antidepressant drugs have been used successfully. In severe cases the patient must be referred to a psychiatrist.

Crenated Tongue

Crenated tongue consists of shallow impressions on the lateral margins of the tongue due to the neighboring teeth (Fig. **138**). The mucosa is usually normal in appearance but may occasionally be red if there is intense friction or pressure against the teeth.

It is frequently found in persons who have the habit of pressing the tongue hard against the teeth or when teeth malposition exists.

Myxedema, acromegaly, amyloidosis, and lipoid proteinosis are diseases that may cause macroglossia and subsequently crenated tongue.

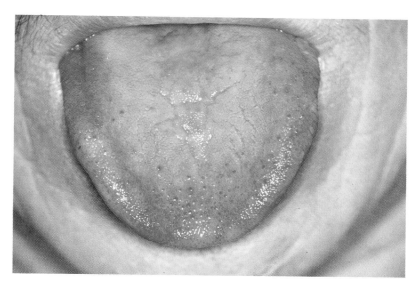

Fig. **136**. Plasma cell glossitis.

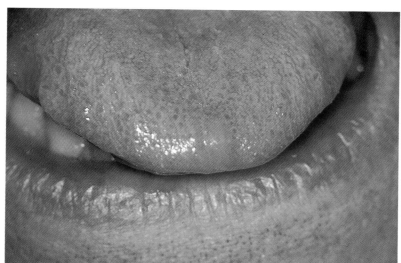

Fig. **137**. Glossodynia, slight erythema and mild elongation of fungiform papillae at the tip of the tongue.

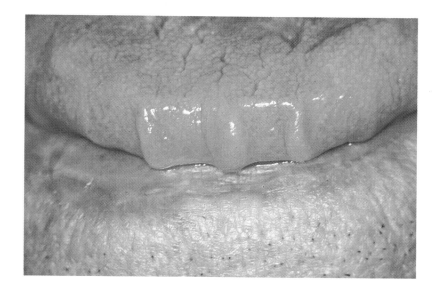

Fig. **138**. Crenated tongue.

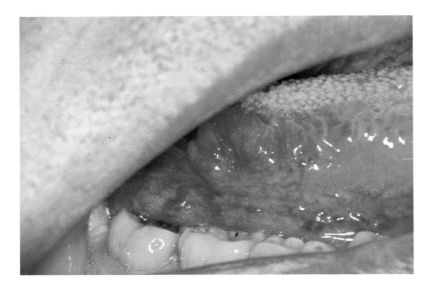

Fig. **139**. Hypertrophy of foliate papillae.

Hypertrophy of Foliate Papillae

The foliate papillae are localized in the posterior lateral borders of the tongue and may be rudimentary in size or they may appear as large protruding nodules.

They may become inflamed and enlarged in response to local chronic irritation or infection (Fig. **139**).

The patient may complain of a burning sensation and frequently be alarmed by the enlarged papillae, fearing a cancer.

Treatment. Reassurance is indicated.

Hypertrophy of Circumvallate Papillae

The circumvallate papillae are located on the posterior aspect of the dorsum of the tongue. They are 8 to 12 in number arranged in a V-shaped pattern. Hypertrophy of the circumvallate papillae results in red, well-circumscribed raised nodules (Fig. **140**), which, when discovered by the patient, may cause fear of a cancer.

Treatment. No treatment is indicated apart from reassurance.

Hypertrophy of the Fungiform Papillae

The fungiform papillae appear as multiple small round red nodules along the anterior portion of the dorsum of the tongue.

Fungiform papillae sometimes become inflamed and enlarged, causing a burning sensation or mild pain, mainly at the tip of the tongue. Excessive smoking, alcohol consumption, hot foods, mechanical friction, irregular tooth surfaces, spices, etc., may predispose to inflammation and enlargement of the fungiform papillae (Fig. **141**). Elimination of these factors is indicated.

Sublingual Varices

In persons more than 60 years of age varicosities of the sublingual veins are common. Clinically, they appear as tortuous, sublingual veins with widened nodule-like areas at the ventral surface and the lateral border of the tongue (Fig. **142**). Sublingual varices are benign and they are usually discovered accidentally by the patient.

Treatment. No therapy except reassurance is required.

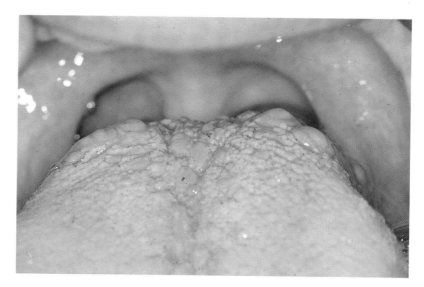

Fig. **140**. Hypertrophy of circumvallate papillae.

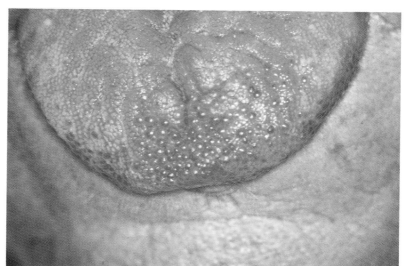

Fig. **141**. Hypertrophy of fungiform papillae.

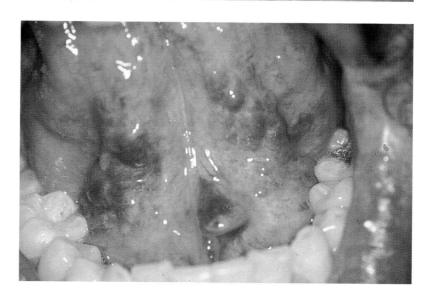

Fig. **142**. Sublingual varices.

13. Diseases of the Lips

Angular Cheilitis

Angular cheilitis, or perlèche, is a disorder of the lips caused by several factors, such as riboflavin deficiency, iron deficiency anemia, Plummer-Vinson syndrome, mechanical trauma. However, many cases are due to loss of proper vertical dimension of the teeth, which may occur in patients who wear dentures or in edentulous persons. In such cases, a fold is formed at the angles of the mouth in which saliva continuously moistens the region, producing maceration and fissuring. It has been shown that microorganisms, such as Candida albicans, Streptococci, Staphylococci, and others may superimpose or cause angular cheilitis. Clinically, the condition is characterized by maceration, fissuring, erythema with erosions, and crusting at the commissures (Fig. **143**). Characteristically, the lesions do not extend beyond the mucocutaneous border. A burning sensation and feeling of dryness may occur. Untreated, angular cheilitis, may last for a long time, showing remissions and exacerbations.

Treatment consists of correction of the occlusal vertical dimension, vitamin administration, and local steroid or antibiotic ointment.

Actinic Cheilitis

Actinic cheilitis may occur as an acute or chronic process. Chronic actinic cheilitis is observed in older persons as a result of long-standing exposure to sunlight (such as farmers, seamen) and characteristically involves the lower lip.

During the early stage, mild edema and slight erythema of the lower lip are common findings, followed by dryness and fine scaling. Progressively, the epithelium becomes thin, atrophic with small whitish-gray areas intermingled with red regions (Fig. **144**). Later, the lip becomes very dry and scaly. Nodules and sometimes erosions may form. There is an increased risk of development of leukoplakia and squamous cell carcinoma.

The differential diagnosis should include lupus erythematosus, lichen planus, contact cheilitis, leukoplakia, and squamous cell carcinoma.

Laboratory test. Histopathologic examination is essential to exclude cancer.

Treatment consists of protection from prolonged exposure to the sun, local application of 5-fluorouracil, and, in severe cases, surgical excision of the involved areas of the lip.

Exfoliative Cheilitis

Exfoliative cheilitis is a chronic inflammatory disorder of the vermilion border of the lips, which is characterized by the persistent formation of scales and crusts. It is most commonly observed in young women with emotional stress and may coexist with atopy. The cause is unknown, although the lesions may become aggravated by cold or very hot weather. Clinically, exfoliative cheilitis consists of severe exfoliation of the vermilion border of the lips leaving an erythematous and sensitive surface. This pattern is repetitive, resulting in thickening, scaling, and crusting of one or both lips (Fig. **145**). Exfoliative cheilitis may persist with variable severity for months or years, with remissions and exacerbations, and may cause a significant cosmetic problem to the patient.

The differential diagnosis includes contact cheilitis and actinic cheilitis.

Treatment. Topical moistening agents (such as cocoa butter) and topical steroids may be helpful.

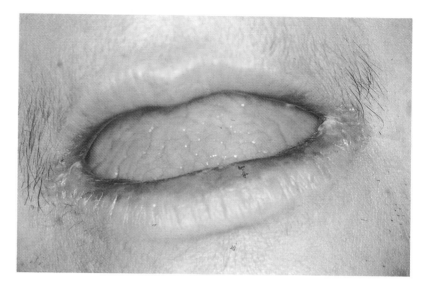

Fig. **143**. Angular cheilitis.

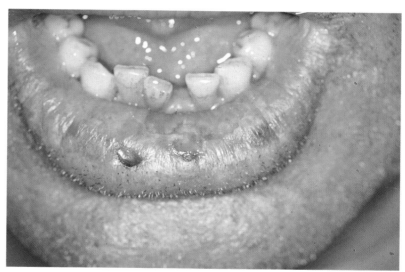

Fig. **144**. Actinic cheilitis.

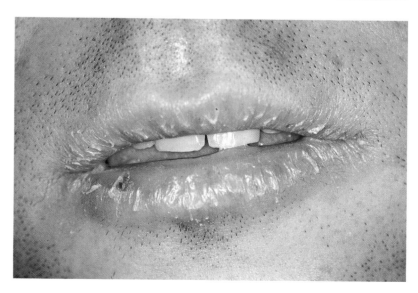

Fig. **145**. Exfoliative cheilitis.

Contact Cheilitis

Contact cheilitis is an inflammatory disorder of the lips that is attributed to allergy to various chemical agents. The most common causes that have been incriminated are lipsticks, lip salves, dentrifices, mouthwashes, foods, etc. Clinically, contact cheilitis is characterized by mild edema and erythema, followed by irritation and scaling (Fig. **146**). It is usually confined to the vermilion border of the lips. A careful history is essential to determine the probable cause. In addition, a patch test is necessary to confirm the causative substance.

The differential diagnosis includes exfoliative cheilitis, and plasma cell cheilitis.

Treatment consists of discontinuing all contact with the offending substance and use of topical steroids.

Cheilitis Glandularis

Cheilitis glandularis is an uncommon chronic inflammatory disorder involving chiefly the lower lip. The cause is unknown, although in some cases a hereditary pattern is observed. Emotional stress and chronic exposure to sunlight have also been incriminated. Clinically, it consists of enlargement of the lip due to minor salivary gland hyperplasia and chronic inflammatory infiltration (Fig. **147**). Characteristically, the orifices of the secretory ducts are dilated and appear as numerous pinhead openings from which mucus or mucopustular fluid may be expressed on pressure. Crusting, erosions, and abscesses may also occur.

Three forms of cheilitis glandularis are recognized: a simple form, which is the most common, a superficial suppurative form, and a deep suppurative form. The last two forms are a result of microbial infection and the clinical signs and symptoms are more severe.

The differential diagnosis includes cheilitis granulomatosa, sarcoidosis, Crohn's disease, lymphangioma, and tuberculosis.

Laboratory test. Histopathologic examination is essential in establishing the diagnosis.

Treatment. Topical steroids are of limited value. In advanced cases plastic surgery is indicated.

Cheilitis Granulomatosa

Cheilitis granulomatosa, or Miescher's cheilitis, is an uncommon chronic disorder of unknown cause. It may occur either as an isolated disorder or as part of several other diseases, such as the Melkersson-Rosenthal syndrome, sarcoidosis, and Crohn's disease. However, the isolated cases are believed to be a monosymptomatic form of the Melkersson-Rosenthal syndrome. Clinically, cheilitis granulomatosa is characterized by painless, diffuse swelling, frequently of the lower lip and rarely the upper lip or both (Fig. **148**). The surrounding skin and oral mucosa may be normal or erythematous. Small vesicles, erosions, and scaling may occasionally appear. The disease usually has a sudden onset and a chronic course, with remissions and exarcerbations, finally leading to permanent enlargement of the lips.

The differential diagnosis includes cheilitis glandularis, sarcoidosis, Crohn's disease, lymphoedema, lymphangioma, erysipelas, and angioneurotic edema.

Laboratory test. Histophatologic examination is essential to establish the diagnosis.

Treatment. Topical steroid ointments, intralesional injection of triamcinolone, or systemic steroids may be useful in some cases. However, in advanced cases plastic surgery is indicated.

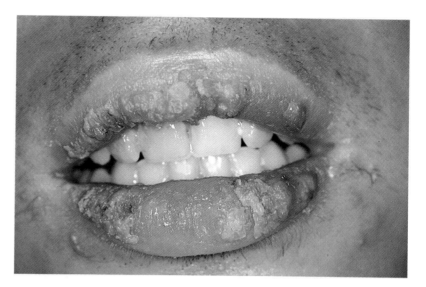

Fig. **146**. Contact cheilitis.

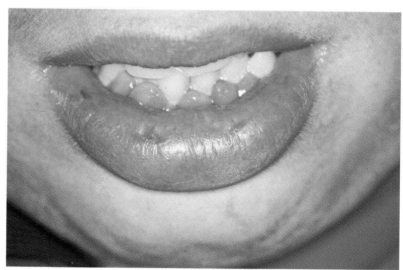

Fig. **147**. Cheilitis glandularis.

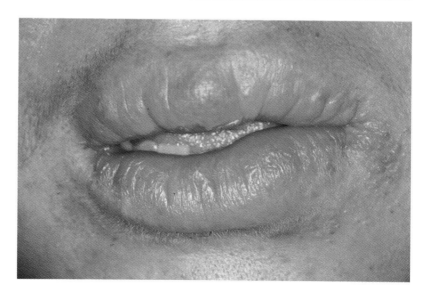

Fig. **148**. Cheilitis granulomatosa.

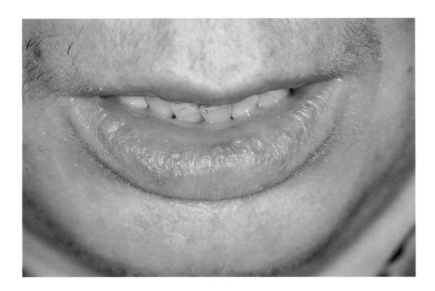

Fig. **149**. Plasma cell cheilitis.

Plasma Cell Cheilitis

Plasma cell cheilitis is an uncommon inflammatory disorder of the lips, characterized by a dense infiltration of mature plasma cells.

The cause remains unknown, and the lesion usually occurs in patients more than 60 years of age. Clinically, it is characterized by diffuse redness with slight swelling of the vermilion border of the lower lip (Fig. **149**). Similar lesions have been described on the gingiva and the tongue. This group of lesions is identical to plasma cell balanitis (Zoon's disease).

The differential diagnosis includes contact cheilitis, allergic reactions, actinic cheilitis, erythroplakia, candidosis, lichen planus, and lupus erythematosus.

Laboratory test. Histopathologic examination is helpful in establishing the diagnosis.

Treatment is symptomatic, and topical steroids may be helpful.

14. Soft Tissue Cysts

Mucocele

Mucoceles, or mucous cysts, originate from minor salivary glands or their ducts and are the most common cysts of the oral soft tissues. Two types are recognized: extravasation mucoceles are most common (more than 80%) and their pathogenesis is related to duct rupture from trauma due to biting; retention mucoceles are rare and their pathogenesis is related to partial obstruction of the duct, probably due to infection, calculus, or sialoliths.

Extravasation-type mucoceles display a peak incidence during the second and third decades, whereas the retention-type mucoceles are more common in older age groups. However, there is no sex predilection, and they may occur at all ages. Most frequently, mucoceles occur on the lower lip, usually laterally, at the level of the bicuspids, less commonly on the buccal mucosa, floor of the mouth, palate, tongue, and very seldom on the upper lip.

Clinically, mucoceles are painless, spherical, solitary fluctuant masses that vary in size from a few millimeters to several centimeters in diameter (Figs. **150, 151**). Superficial cysts are translucent and bluish, whereas deeper lesions have the color of normal mucosa. Usually, they appear suddenly, rapidly reaching their final size, and may persist for several weeks to several months. Sometimes they empty partially and then reform due to accumulation of fresh fluid.

The differential diagnosis includes hemangioma, lymphangioma, lipoma, papillary cystadenoma lymphomatosum, mucoepidermoid tumor, and Sjögren's syndrome.

Laboratory test. Histopathologic examination is useful in establishing the diagnosis.

Treatment consists of surgical excision or cryosurgery.

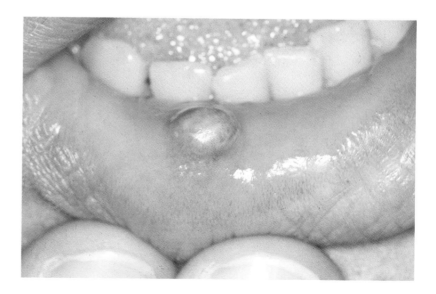

Fig. **150**. Mucocele of the lower lip.

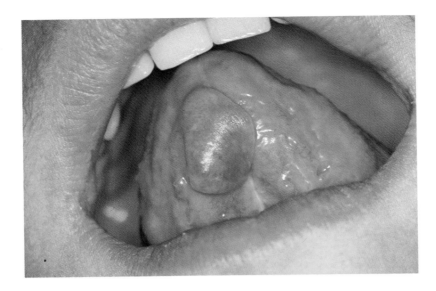

Fig. **151**. Mucocele of the tongue.

Ranula

Ranula is a variety of mucocele localized exlusively in the floor of the mouth. It arises from the ducts of the submandibular gland, sublingual gland, or the accessory salivary glands of the floor of the mouth, and its pathogenesis is similar to that of mucoceles. Clinically, it presents as a smooth, fluctuant, painless mass in the floor of the mouth, just lateral to the lingual frenum (Fig. **152**). The color ranges from normal to translucent bluish.

The average size is 1 to 2 cm, but larger lesions may form, causing speech and swallowing problems.

The differential diagnosis includes dermoid cyst, lymphoepithelial cyst, abscess of the floor of the mouth, hemangioma, lymphangioma, etc.

Laboratory test. Histopathologic examination establishes the diagnosis.

Treatment consists of surgical removal.

Lymphoepithelial Cyst

Lymphoepithelial cyst of the oral mucosa is an uncommon developmental lesion that is probably due to cystic degeneration of glandular epithelium entrapped within oral lymphoid tissue during embryogenesis. It usually becomes apparent between the ages of 20 and 50 years and is slightly more frequent in men than women (ratio 3:2). Intraoral lymphoepithelial cyst is histologically similar to the branchial cleft cyst that develops in the neck. The intraoral cyst occurs most frequently in the floor of the mouth and the ventral surface of the tongue, although sporadic cases have been described in other sites. Clinically, it is a mobile, painless, well-defined, firm, and elevated nodule with a yellowish or reddish color (Fig. **153**). The size ranges from a few millimeters to 2 cm in diameter.

The differential diagnosis includes lymph node, dermoid cyst, mucocele, lipoma, and other benign tumors.

Laboratory test. Histopathologic examination is essential to establish the diagnosis.

Treatment is surgical removal.

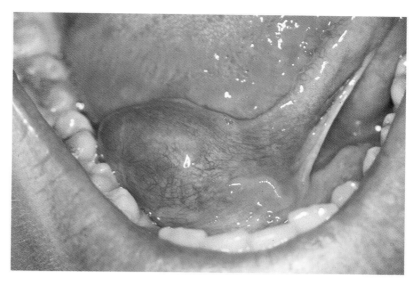

Fig. **152**. Ranula.

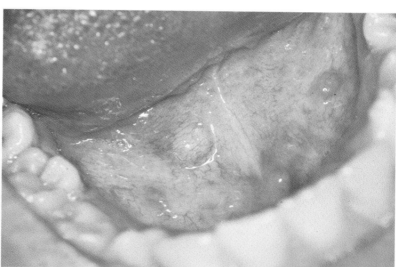

Fig. **153**. Lymphoepithelial cyst in the floor of the mouth.

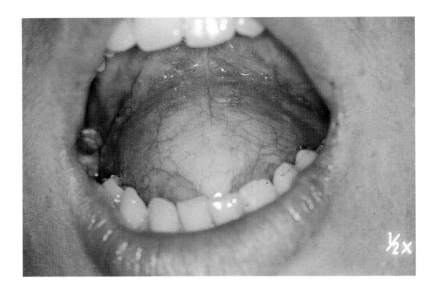

Fig. **154**. Dermoid cyst.

Dermoid Cyst

Dermoid cyst is an uncommon developmental lesion arising from embryonic epithelial remnants. Dermoid cyst of the oral cavity is usually situated in the midline of the floor of the mouth. The cyst frequently appears in early adulthood and both sexes are equally affected. The size is small, but the cyst progressivelly and slowly expands and finally may reach several centimeters in diameter. Clinically, it is a painless elevated swelling with normal or slightly reddish color and characteristic soft doughlike consistency on palpation (Fig. **154**). When the cyst is located above the geniohyoid muscle, it displaces the tongue upward, producing difficulties in mastication, speech, and swallowing. If located between the geniohyoid and mylohyoid muscles, it protrudes submentally.

The differential diagnosis includes lymphoepithelial cyst, ranula, cystic hygroma, and abscess of the floor of the mouth.

Laboratory test. Histopathologic examination is essential for the final diagnosis.

Treatment is surgical removal.

Eruption Cyst

Eruption cyst is a variety of dentigerous cyst that is associated with an erupting deciduous or permanent tooth. It is commonly located at the site of eruption of the canines and molars. Clinically, eruption cyst appears as a well-demarcated, fluc-

tuant, and soft swelling directly overlying the alveolus at the site of the erupting tooth. Very often, the color is blue, or dark red when the cyst cavity is filled with blood (Figs. **155, 156**). The clinical features are characteristic and the diagnosis is obvious.

The differential diagnosis includes hemangioma, hematoma, amalgam tattoo, oral pigmented nevi, and malignant melanoma.

Laboratory test. Histopathologic examination confirms the diagnosis.

Treatment usually is not required. However, the soft tissue cap may be excised.

Gingival Cyst of the Newborn

Gingival cysts of the newborn, or Epstein's pearls or Bohn's nodules, are small lesions on the alveolar ridge of newborn infants. It arises from remmants of the dental lamina. Clinically, it appears as multiple or solitary asymptomatic whitish nodules 1 to 3 mm in diameter in the alveolar mucosa (Fig. **157**). These cysts contain keratin and regress spontaneously within a few months.

The differential diagnosis includes lymphangioma.

Laboratory test. Histopathologic examination confirms the diagnosis.

Treatment is not required.

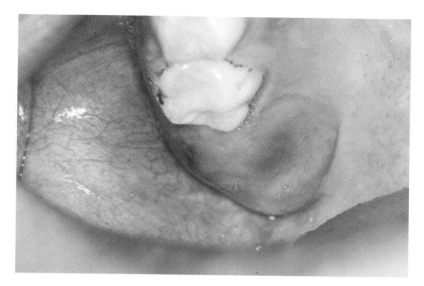

Fig. **155**. Eruption cyst.

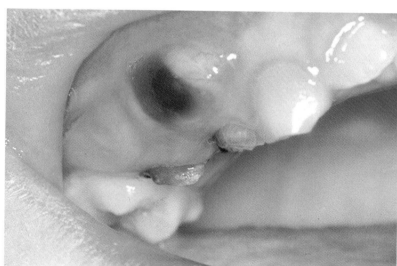

Fig. **156**. Eruption cyst.

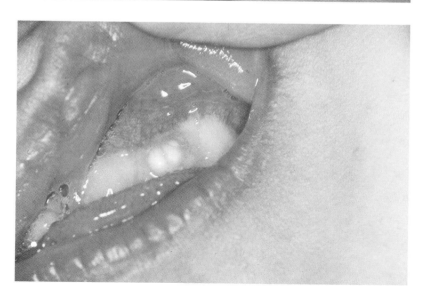

Fig. **157**. Gingival cyst of the new-born.

Gingival Cyst of the Adult

Gingival cyst is rare in adult patients and may be located either in the free or attached gingiva. It originates from epithelial rests (such as dental lamina) in the gingiva. It is more frequent in patients more than 40 years of age and is located most often to the mandibular vestibule between the lateral incisor and first premolar. Clinically, it appears as a small well-circumscribed nodule of the gingiva, covered with normal mucosa with a size varying from few millimeters to 1 cm in diameter (Fig. **158**).

The differential diagnosis includes mucocele, periodontal abscess, peripheral ossifying fibroma, and traumatic fibroma.

Laboratory test. Histopathologic examination is essential in establishing the diagnosis.

Treatment is surgical excision.

Palatine Papilla Cyst

Palatine papilla cyst is a variety of the naso-palatine cyst that arises from epithelial rests in the incisive foramen. Clinically, it appears as a soft swelling of the palatine papilla, covered with normal mucosa (Fig. **159**). Often, it may become inflamed and painful due to infection. On radiographic examination, there are no pathologic findings.

The differential diagnosis includes dental and periodontal abscess, trauma of the palatine papilla, fibroma, and other benign tumors of the oral connective tissue.

Laboratory test. Histopathologic examination is necessary to establish the diagnosis.

Treatment is surgical removal.

Thyroglossal Duct Cyst

Thyroglossal duct cyst is a rare developmental lesion that may form anywhere along the thyroglossal duct from the foramen caecum of the tongue to the thyroid glands. It is more frequent in younger persons and appears as a firm circumscribed midline cystic swelling a few millimeters to several centimeters in diameter. When it is localized in the oral cavity, it is usually found on the dorsum of the tongue close to the foramen caecum (Fig. **160**). On rare occasions, it may be found in the floor of the mouth. It grows slowly and, if significantly enlarged, may cause dysphagia. A fistula may form on occasion, opening on the skin or mucosal surface.

The differential diagnosis includes benign and malignant tumors and median rhomboid glossitis.

Laboratory test. Histopathologic examination is necessary to establish the diagnosis.

Treatment is surgical excision.

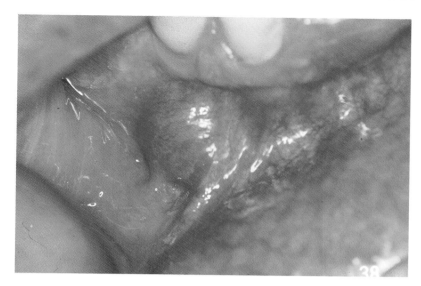

Fig. **158**. Gingival cyst of the adults.

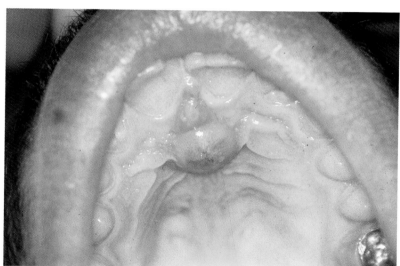

Fig. **159**. Palatine papilla cyst.

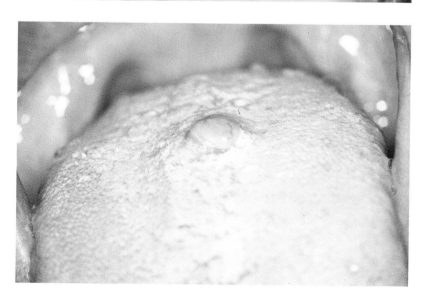

Fig. **160**. Thyroglossal duct cyst on the dorsum of the tongue.

15. Viral Infections

Primary Herpetic Gingivostomatitis

Primary herpetic gingivostomatitis is the most frequent acute viral infection of the oral mucosa. It mainly affects children and young adults. The cause of the disease is the herpes simplex virus, type 1 (HSV-1). Primary contact with the HSV-1 may produce either acute primary disease or a subclinical asymptomatic infection: both lead to immunity. Clinically, primary herpetic gingivostomatitis is characterized by high temperature, malaise, irritability, headache, pain in the mouth, followed within 1 to 3 days by the eruptive phase. The oral mucosa is red and edematous, with numerous coalescing vesicles. Within 24 hours, the vesicles rupture, leaving painful small, round, shallow ulcers covered by a yellowish-gray pseudomembrane and surrounded by an erythematous halo (Fig. 161). New elements continue to appear during the first 3 to 5 days. The ulcers gradually heal in 10 to 14 days without scarring. Bilateral painful regional lymphadenopathy is a constant feature of the disease. Lesions are almost always present on the gingiva, resulting in acute gingivitis, which may be free of vesicles (Fig. 162). Any other area of the oral mucosa may also be affected, that is, the buccal mucosa, tongue, lips, and palate. The oral lesions are usually scattered, although solitary lesions may be seen.

The diagnosis is based on the clinical features and only rarely is laboratory confirmation required.

The differential diagnosis includes herpetiform ulcers, aphthous ulcers, hand-foot-and-mouth disease, herpangina, streptococcal stomatitis, acute necrotizing ulcerative gingivitis, erythema multiforme, and pemphigus vulgaris.

Laboratory test. Cytologic examination is definitive for intranuclear viral infection. Histopathologic studies, monoclonal antibodies, isolation, and culture of the virus (nucleic acid hybridization) confirm the diagnosis in difficult cases. An elevated serum titer of antibodies is also suggestive of the disease.

Treatment. In severe cases acyclovir systemically is indicated, but in most cases treatment is symptomatic.

Secondary Herpetic Stomatitis

Reactivation of HSV-1 in preinfected persons may cause recurrent intraoral herpes simplex.

Recurrent herpes infection differs from primary infection in that the vesicles are closely grouped, smaller in size, and the constitutional symptoms are absent. Predisposing factors that may precipitate reactivation of the virus include emotional stress, febrile illness, needle trauma after an oral injection, and extraction of a tooth. In addition, recently it has been recorded that recurrent herpetic lesions is a common manifestation in acquired immune deficiency syndrome (AIDS-related complex and AIDS patients).

The clinical features consist of a small number of discrete vesicles arranged in clusters, usually localized on the hard palate and the attached gingiva. The vesicles rupture in a few hours, leaving small, 1 to 3 mm ulcers that heal spontaneously in 6 to 10 days without scarring (Fig. 163).

Because of acquired immunity during the primary infection, the subjective complaints are usually mild and constitutional symptoms are characteristically absent. The diagnosis is made exclusively on clinical criteria.

The differential diagnosis includes herpetiform ulcers, aphthous ulcers, herpes zoster, streptococcal stomatitis, gonococcal stomatitis, primary and secondary syphilis.

Treatment is symptomatic.

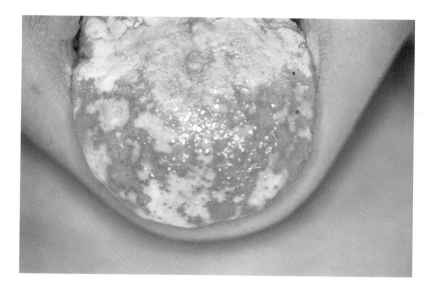

Fig. **161**. Primary herpetic gingivo-stomatitis, multiple ulcers on the tongue.

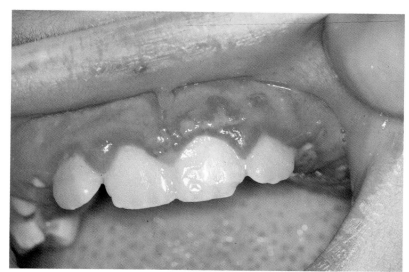

Fig. **162**. Primary herpetic gingivo-stomatitis, erythema and multiple ulcers on the gingiva.

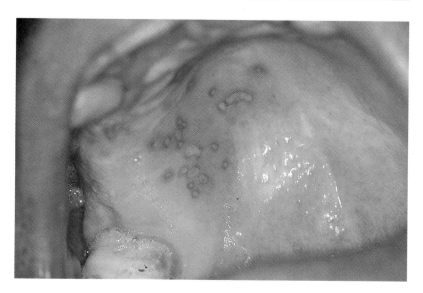

Fig. **163**. Secondary herpetic stomatitis, round small ulcers on the palate.

Herpes Labialis

Herpes labialis is due to reactivation of HSV-1 from its location in nerve ganglia, and it is by far the most common form of recurrent herpetic infection. It affects women more often than men in a ratio of about 2:1 and involves the upper or lower lip with equal frequency. Prodromal symptoms, such as burning, mild pain, and itching, usually precede the eruption by a few hours. Clinically, it is characterized by edema and redness on the vermilion border and the adjacent perioral skin, followed by clusters of small vesicles.

The vesicles soon rupture, leaving small ulcers that are covered by crusts and heal spontaneously in 5 to 8 days (Fig. **164**).

Frequently, recurrences may be associated with fever, emotional stress, menstruation, light exposure, cold weather, mechanical trauma, etc. The diagnosis is made usually on clinical grounds.

The differential diagnosis includes traumatic lesions, primary and secondary syphilis, and impetigo.

Treatment is symptomatic and is strengthened by topical application of acyclovir.

Herpes Zoster

Herpes zoster is an acute localized viral disease caused by reactivation of a latent varicella-zoster virus. Herpes zoster affects elderly persons, usually more than 50 years old, and is rare in infants and children. An increased incidence of herpes zoster occurs in Hodgkin's disease, leukemias and other cancers, AIDS, after administration of corticosteroids and other immunosuppressive drugs, and during radiation therapy. The thoracic, cervical, trigeminal, and lumbosacral dermatomes are most frequently affected. Clinically, the first manifestation of the disease is usually tenderness and pain in the involved dermatome. Constitutional symptoms, such as fever, malaise, and headache may also occur. After 2 to 4 days, the eruptive phase follows, characterized by grouped maculopapules on an erythematous base, which rapidly form vesicles and in 2 to 3 days evolve into pustules. Within 5 to 10 days, the pustules crust and persist for 10 to 20 days. New lesions continue to appear for several days. The regional lymph nodes are usually tender and enlarged. The unilateral location of the lesions is the most characteristic clinical feature of herpes zoster. Oral manifestations may occur when the second and third branchs of the trigeminal nerve are involved. Frequently, intraoral involvement is associated with unilateral skin lesions on the face. Oral mucosal lesions are almost identical to the cutaneous lesions. An itching sensation and pain, which may simulate pulpitis, precede oral lesions. These begin as unilateral clusters of vesicles, which in 2 to 3 days rupture, leaving ulcers surrounded by a broad erythematous zone (Figs. **165, 166**). The ulcers heal without scarring in 2 to 3 weeks. Postherpetic trigeminal neuralgia is the most common complication of oral herpes zoster. Rarely, osteomyelitis, necrosis of the jaw bone, or loss of teeth may occur in immunocompromised patients.

The diagnosis of oral herpes zoster is based on clinical criteria.

The differential diagnosis should consider secondary herpetic stomatitis.

Laboratory test. Cytologic examination confirms virally modified epithelial cells.

Treatment is symptomatic. Analgesics and sedatives may help to control the pain. Low-dose corticosteroids (such as 20 to 30 mg prednisolone per day) during the early stage of the disease may reduce the possibility of postherpetic neuralgia. Acyclovir and other antiviral agents may be helpful in severe cases.

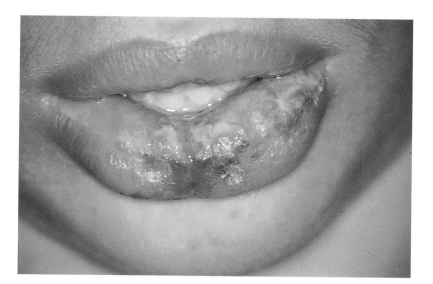

Fig. **164**. Herpes labialis.

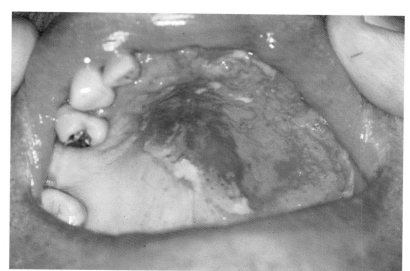

Fig. **165**. Herpes zoster affecting the left side of the palate.

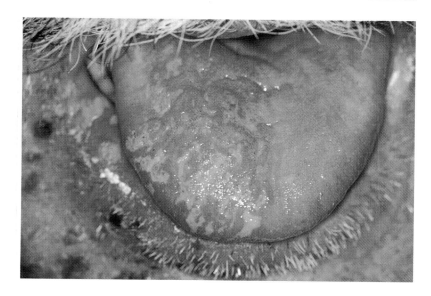

Fig. **166**. Herpes zoster affecting the right side of the tongue.

Varicella

Varicella (chickenpox) is an acute exanthematous and highly contagious disease of childhood caused by primary infection with the varicella-zoster virus. The disease shows an increased prevalence in winter and spring. An incubation period of 10 to 20 days is common, followed by headache, low-grade fever, and a maculopapular skin rash that rapidly becomes vesicular, pustular, and finally crusting. New elements appear in successive waves over 2 to 4 days and the presence of lesions at different stages is a characteristic clinical feature. The trunk, face, and scalp are most commonly involved.

In the oral mucosa a few small vesicles appear that soon rupture, leaving erosions with a whitish surface and red halo (Fig. **167**). Oral lesions are common and show a predilection for the palate and the lips. Vesicles may also appear on other mucous membranes.

The diagnosis is made on clinical grounds.

The differential diagnosis of oral lesions includes herpetic lesions, aphthous ulcer, and streptococcal stomatitis.

Treatment is symptomatic.

Herpangina

Herpangina is a specific acute infection caused by Coxsackie virus group A, types 1–6, 8, 10, and 22 and occasionally other types. It has a peak incidence during summer and autumn and frequently affects children and young adults. Clinically, the disease presents with sudden fever (ranging from 38° to 40°C), sore throat, headache, dysphagia, and malaise followed within 24 to 48 hours by diffuse erythema and a vesicular eruption of the posterior oral mucosa and oropharynx.

The vesicles are numerous, small, and soon rupture, leaving painful shallow ulcers that heal in 7 to 10 days (Fig. **168**). The lesions characteristically involve the soft palate and uvula, the tonsils, faucial pillars, posterior pharyngeal wall, and rarely the buccal mucosa and the tongue.

The absence of lesions from the lips, gingiva, and the floor of the mouth are characteristic. The disease lasts for 7 to 12 days, and the diagnosis is exclusively based on clinical criteria.

The differential diagnosis includes primary herpetic gingivostomatitis, aphthous ulcers, herpetiform ulcers, acute lymphonodular pharyngitis, streptococcal and gonococcal pharyngitis, and erythema multiforme.

Laboratory tests to confirm the diagnosis are the isolation of the virus and serology, although they are not usually needed.

Treatment is symptomatic.

Acute Lymphonodular Pharyngitis

Acute lymphonodular pharyngitis is an acute febrile disease caused by Coxsackie virus A10.

The disease frequently affects children and young adults. Clinically, it presents with fever (ranging from 38° to 41°C), a mild headache, anorexia, and sore throat, followed within 2 to 3 days by a characteristic nonvesicular eruption on the uvula, soft palate, anterior tonsillar pillars, and posterior pharynx (Fig. **169**). The lesions consist of multiple, raised, discrete papules whitish to yellowish in color surrounded by an erythematous halo. The size of the lesions vary from 3 to 6 mm in diameter and they last 4 to 8 days.

The differential diagnosis includes herpangina and herpes simplex.

Laboratory tests to confirm the diagnosis are the isolation of the virus and serologic examination.

Treatment is symptomatic and the disease is self-limiting.

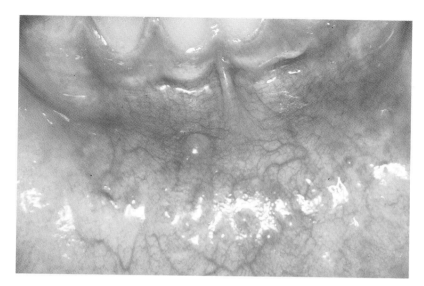

Fig. **167**. Varicella, small vesicle on the lower lip mucosa.

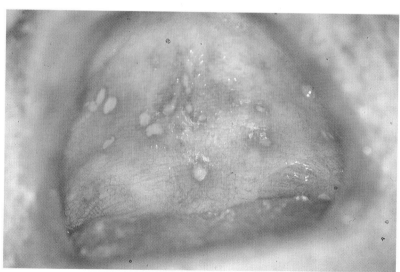

Fig. **168**. Herpangina, numerous shallow ulcers on the soft palate.

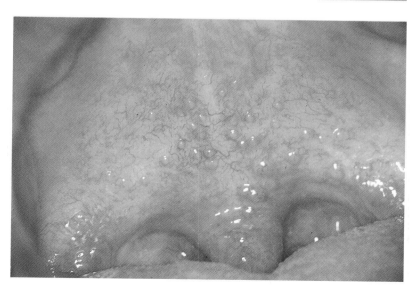

Fig. **169**. Acute lymphonodular pharyngitis, multiple discrete papules on the soft palate and uvula.

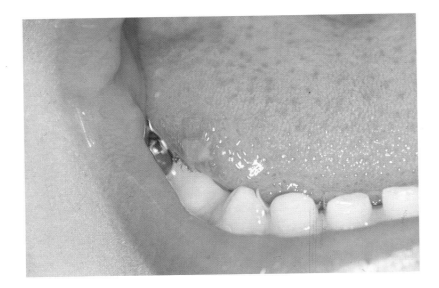

Fig. **170**. Hand-foot-and-mouth disease, shallow ulcer on the tongue.

Hand-Foot-and-Mouth Disease

Hand-foot-and-mouth disease is usually associated with Coxsackie virus A16, occasionally with A5, A10, and infrequently with other types. It usually affects children and young adults. The disease may occur in epidemics or isolated cases. Clinically, there appear a few (5 to 10 in number) small vesicles that soon rupture, leaving slightly painful, shallow ulcers (2 to 6 mm in diameter) surrounded by a red halo (Fig. **170**). The tongue, buccal mucosa, and palate are the usual sites of involvement. Skin lesions are inconstant, and small vesicles surrounded by a narrow red halo are present. The lateral and dorsal surfaces of the fingers and toes are the more frequently involved areas (Figs. **171, 172**). However, lesions may occur on the palms, soles, and buttocks. Low-grade fever of short duration and malaise may be present. The disease lasts 5 to 8 days.

The diagnosis is based on clinical criteria.

The differential diagnosis includes aphthous ulcers, herpetiform ulcers, primary and secondary herpetic stomatitis, and herpangina.

Laboratory test. Isolation of the virus and inoculation in newborn mice may be needed to confirm the diagnosis in atypical cases.

Treatment is supportive.

Measles

Measles is an acute, contagious infection of childhood, caused by a specific paramyxovirus. After an incubation period of 8 to 12 days the patient presents with fever, malaise, chills, cough, and conjunctivitis. Three to 4 days later a characteristic maculopapular rash appears behind the ears and on the forehead and spreads within 24 hours to the rest of the face, the neck, the trunk, and the extremities. The rash fades from the 6th to 10th days. Characteristic bluish-white specks with bright red areola (Koplik's spots) may appear on the buccal mucosa at the level of the first and second molars, 1 to 2 days before onset of the rash. Koplik's spots are transient and usually absent. A diffuse erythema, petechiae, and rarely small round erosions on the oral mucosa may also be observed (Fig. **173**). Complications are encephalitis, otitis media, pneumonia, and enteritis.

The differential diagnosis of oral lesions includes acute candidosis, minor aphthous ulcers, herpetic lesions, infectious mononucleosis, and varicella.

Laboratory test. Serologic tests are useful in the diagnosis of atypical cases.

Treatment is symptomatic.

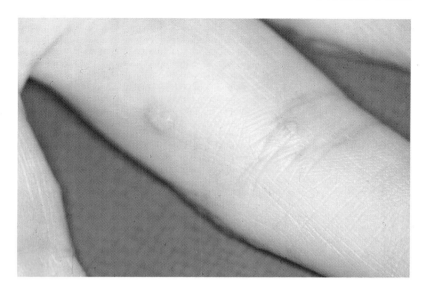

Fig. **171**. Hand-foot-and-mouth disease, two small vesicles on the fingers.

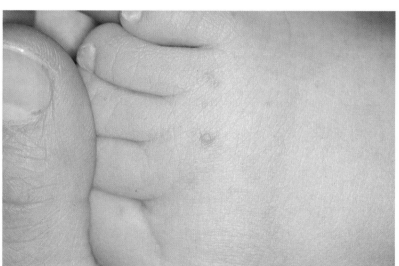

Fig. **172**. Hand-foot-and-mouth disease, small vesicles on the foot.

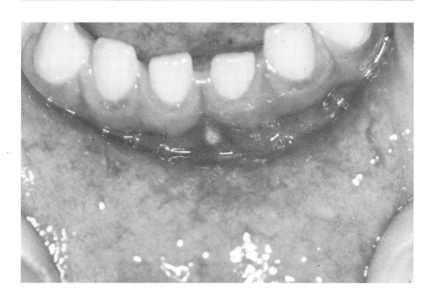

Fig. **173**. Measles, small erosion on the mucolabial fold.

Infectious Mononucleosis

Infectious mononucleosis is an acute self-limited disease caused by the Epstein-Barr virus. The virus is frequently transmitted through salivary transfer. Infectious mononucleosis is more common in children and young adults. The incubation period is about 30 to 50 days, followed by low-grade fever, which persists for 1 to 2 weeks, malaise, mild headache, and fatigue. Generalized lymphadenopathy also begins early and is a common manifestation. Splenomegaly, hepatomegaly, and very rarely central nervous system involvement may also occur. A maculopapular eruption usually on the trunk and arms is present in 5 to 15% of cases. The oral manifestations are early and frequent, and the most constant features are palatal petechiae, uvular edema, tonsillar exudate, diffuse erythema of the oral mucosa, gingivitis, and rarely ulcers (Fig. **174**). Sore throat, tonsillitis, and pharyngitis may also occur in association with the oral lesions.

The diagnosis is usually based on the clinical features.

The differential diagnosis of oral lesions includes lesions from fellatio, streptococcal oropharyngitis, diphtheria, leukemia, and secondary syphilis.

Laboratory tests. The diagnosis is confirmed by heterophile antibody tests and other specific antibody tests.

Treatment is symptomatic.

Verruca Vulgaris

Verruca vulgaris, or common wart, is a benign skin lesion caused by a specific human papilloma virus. The most prevalent sites of localization are the backs of the fingers and the hands. From these lesions, the virus may be autoinoculated to the oral mucosa.

Verruca vulgaris is relatively uncommon in the oral mucosa and is clinically and histologically similar to its cutaneous counterpart. Clinically, it appears as a small sessile, well-defined exophytic growth with a cauliflower surface and whitish or normal color (Fig. **175**). The oral lesions may be single or multiple and are frequently located on the lips, palate, and rarely in other oral regions.

The differential diagnosis includes papilloma, condyloma acuminatum, early verrucous carcinoma, and verruciform xanthoma.

Laboratory test. Histopathologic examination confirms the diagnosis.

Treatment consists of surgical excision.

Condyloma Acuminatum

Condyloma acuminatum, or genital wart, is a common benign virus-induced lesion mainly occurring in the anogenital area. The disease is sexually transmitted and is caused by a human papillomavirus.

Condyloma acuminatum of the oral mucosa is rarely encountered and may be due to autoinoculation from genital condyloma acuminatum or during orogenital contact. An increased incidence of the lesions have been reported in patients infected with the human immunodeficiency virus (HIV). Clinically, it appears as single or multiple small sessile or pedunculated nodules that may proliferate and coalesce, forming cauliflower-like growths (Fig. **176**). The lesions have whitish or normal color and display a tendency to recur. The dorsum of the tongue, gingiva, buccal mucosa, especially near the commissure, and the palate are the sites most commonly affected.

The differential diagnosis includes verruca vulgaris, papilloma, verrucous carcinoma, verruciform xanthoma, molluscum contagiosum, and focal dermal hypoplasia syndrome.

Laboratory test. Histopathologic examination is necessary to confirm the diagnosis.

Treatment consists of surgical excision or electrocautery.

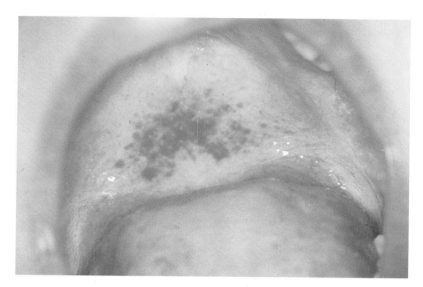

Fig. **174**. Infectious mononucleosis, petechiae on the palate.

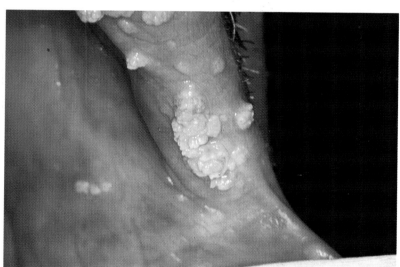

Fig. **175**. Verruca vulgaris, multiple lesions on the lip mucosa.

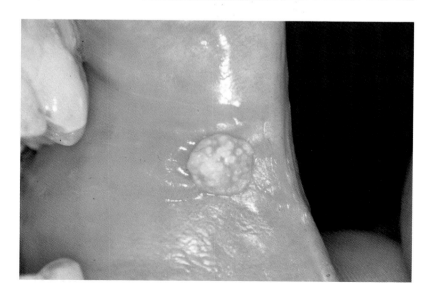

Fig. **176**. Condyloma acuminatum on the buccal mucosa.

Molluscum Contagiosum

Molluscum contagiosum is a benign lesion usually seen on the skin and caused by a pox virus. The lesions may develop at any age, but the majority of cases are found in children. Males are affected more frequently than females. Clinically, the lesions are characterized by grouped, minute, dome-shaped papules, often with central umbilication. Small amounts of whitish fluid may exude on pressure from these lesions. Any skin region may be involved, but the head, eyelids, trunk, and genitalia are most often affected. Molluscum contagiosum is extremely rare in the oral cavity. The clinical picture of oral lesions is similar to the skin lesions and is characterized by multiple small hemispheric papules with a central umbilication (Fig. **177**). The buccal mucosa, labial mucosa, and palate are the sites of involvement in the reported cases.

The differential diagnosis of oral lesions should include lymphangioma, hemangioma, pyogenic granuloma, and condyloma acuminatum.

Laboratory test. Histopathologic examination establishes the final diagnosis.

Treatment. Surgical excision or cryotherapy are the preferred modes of treatment of oral lesions.

Focal Epithelial Hyperplasia

Focal epithelial hyperplasia is a benign hyperplastic lesion of the oral mucosa. It frequently occurs in Eskimos, North American Indians and South Africans, but it has also been reported in other racial groups. Sporadic cases have also been encountered among Europeans and Asians. The causative agent is a human papillomavirus (HPV-13). However, the familial occurrence and the predilection of the disease for certain age groups suggest that a genetic factor could also contribute to the appearance of the lesions. Clinically, it is characterized by multiple painless, sessile, slightly elevated soft papules or nodules 1 to 10 mm in diameter (Figs. **178, 179**). The lesions are whitish or have normal color and smooth surface. On stretching the mucosa, the lesions tend to disappear. The disease is more common in children and the lesions frequently are located on the lower lip, the buccal mucosa, the tongue, and less often on the upper lip, the gingiva, and the palate.

The differential diagnosis includes multiple condylomata acuminata and verruca vulgaris, multiple papillomas and fibromas, Cowden's disease, and focal dermal hypoplasia syndrome.

Laboratory test. Histopathologic examination is essential for diagnosis.

Treatment is nonspecific and should be conservative, since the lesions may disappear within a few months or they may become inactive.

16. Bacterial Infections

Acute Necrotizing Ulcerative Gingivitis

Acute necrotizing ulcerative gingivitis chiefly affects young persons. Although the precise causative agents are unknown, fusiform bacillus, Borrelia vincentii, and other anaerobic microorganisms seem to play an important role. In addition, host factors, such as emotional stress, tobacco use, poor oral hygiene, and local trauma, have been implicated as predisposing factors. Interestingly, acute necrotizing ulcerative gingivitis has been observed among human immunodeficiency virus (HIV)-infected patients. The onset of the disease is either sudden or insidious, and it is clinically characterized by ulceration and necrosis of the interdental papillae and the free margins of the gingiva, which are covered with a dirty yellow-grayish smear (Fig. 191). The gingiva is fiery red, swollen, and extremely painful. The characteristic clinical feature is necrosis of the gingival margins and interdental papillae and the formation of a crater. Spontaneous hemorrhage, intense salivation, and halitosis are common. The disease is usually accompanied by regional lymphadenopathy, fever, and malaise. The lesions may be localized or generalized. The diagnosis may be established on clinical grounds alone.

The differential diagnosis includes primary herpetic gingivostomatitis, streptococcal gingivostomatitis, scurvy, leukemia, and agranulocytosis.

Laboratory test. Smear and histopathologic examination may be helpful sometimes.

Treatment. In the acute phase metronidazole or antibiotics active against anaerobic bacteria are beneficial. Mouthwashes with oxygen-releasing compounds may also be used. Management of the underlying gingivitis must follow the acute phase.

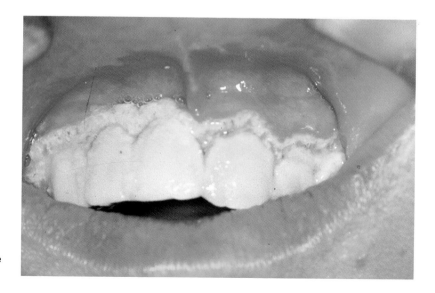

Fig. **191**. Acute necrotizing ulcerative gingivitis.

Acute Necrotizing Ulcerative Stomatitis

Acute necrotizing ulcerative gingivitis may on occasion extend beyond the gingiva and involve other areas of the oral mucosa, usually the buccal mucosa opposite the third molar. Rarely, it may involve the tongue, lips, and palate. Clinically, the oral mucosa is red, ulcerated, with irregular margins, and may be covered with a dirty white-grayish smear (Fig. **192**). In these cases the subjective complaints and objective general phenomena may be more intense.

Cancrum Oris

Cancrum oris, or noma, is a rare but very serious destructive disease usually involving the oral tissues. It more commonly affects children and rarely adults in Africa, Asia, and South America. It is extremely rare in Europe and North America. Vincent's spirochete is always present in the lesions. Predisposing factors include poor oral hygiene, severe protein malnutrition, parasitic diseases, diabetes mellitus, leukemia, and immune defects. Clinically, cancrum oris frequently starts as an ulcerative gingivitis that very soon spreads to the neighboring tissues. Gangrenous necrosis involves the cheeks, lips, and the underlying bone, producing catastrophic lesions of the face (Fig. **193**). The gangrenous ulcers are covered with whitish-brown fibrin and debris. Salivation, halitosis, and fever are always present.

The differential diagnosis includes lethal midline granuloma, malignant tumors, leukemia, and agranulocytosis.

Treatment. Without treatment, the disease is frequently fatal. Antibiotics and a nutritious diet as soon as possible are important. Surgical removal of the destructed tissues is also indicated.

Streptococcal Gingivostomatitis

Streptococcal gingivostomatitis is a debatable disease caused by β-hemolytic Streptococcus. It is a rare entity and the etiologic role of streptococci is controversial because it is not clear whether streptococcal infection is the primary cause or whether it represents a secondary infection of preexisting lesions. The disease is usually localized on the gingiva and rarely in other oral areas (Fig. **194**). Frequently, the oral lesions follow a tonsillitis or upper respiratory infection and are manifested by redness, edema of the gingiva, and patchy superficial, round, or linear erosions covered with a white-yellowish smear. The interdental papillae remain intact. The disease is localized and rarely involves the entire gingival tissues. Mild fever and submandibular lymphadenopathy are also present.

The differential diagnosis includes herpetic gingivostomatitis and acute necrotizing ulcerative gingivitis.

Laboratory test. Gram's stain and isolation of streptococci establishes the diagnosis.

Treatment consists of oral antibiotics, such as penicillin, ampicillin, and erythromycin.

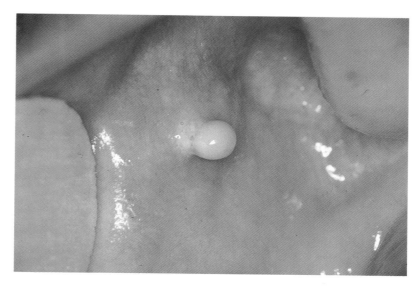

Fig. **198**. Acute suppurative parotitis, pus discharges from the parotid duct opening.

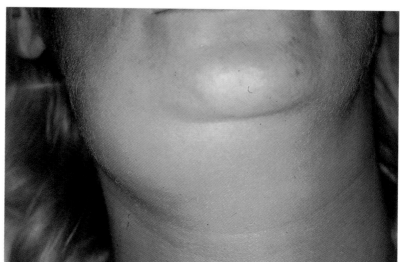

Fig. **199**. Acute submandibular sialadenitis, swelling under the angle and the body of the mandible.

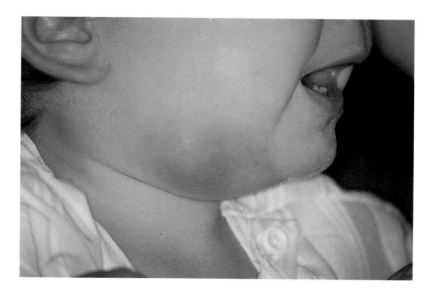

Fig. **200**. Buccal cellulitis, ill-defined erythematous swelling on the skin of the face of a 2-year-old girl.

Syphilis

Syphilis is a venereal disease caused by Treponema pallidum.

Acquired syphilis is most often transmitted through sexual intercourse, but rarely nonvenereal transmission may occur. Placental transmission of T. pallidum from an infected mother to fetus causes congenital syphilis.

The modern classification of syphilis is based on epidemiologic, clinical, and therapeutic criteria, as follows: early syphilis, includes primary and secondary stages and clinical relapses due to incomplete treatment and lasts less than 1 year; latent syphilis, which is subclassified into early stage (lasts less than 2 years) and late stage (lasts 2 years or more); and late syphilis, includes tertiary syphilis, that is, gumma, central nervous system, and cardiovascular manifestations, and lasts 5 or more years.

Primary Syphilis

The primary lesion of acquired syphilis is the chancre. It is usually localized on the genitalia, but in about 10% of the cases the chancre occurs extragenitally (anus, rectum, fingers, nipples, etc.) and especially in the oral cavity. Direct orogenital contact (fellatio or cunnilingus) is the usual mode of transmission of an oral chancre, but kissing may also be responsible if one of the partners has infectious oral lesions.

After an incubation period of 10 to 90 days (average, 21 days), the chancre appears at the site of inoculation.

In males, most chancres tend to appear on the upper lip, and in females, on the lower lip. The tongue is the next most frequent site of involvement, followed by the palate and tonsillar areas. Clinically, the chancre begins as an inflammatory papule that soon erodes. The classic chancre appears as a painless ulcer with a smooth surface, raised border, and indurated base. It is often surrounded by a narrow red border and is covered by a grayish serous exudate teeming with T. pallidum (Figs. **201, 202**).

The chancre is usually solitary, although multiple lesions may appear simultaneously or in rapid succession. It varies in size from a few millimeters to 3 cm in diameter. A constant finding is the enlargement of the regional lymph nodes, which is usually unilateral, less often bilateral. The enlarged lymph nodes are discrete, mobile, hard, and nontender. Without treatment, the chancre heals spontaneously within 3 to 8 weeks.

The diagnosis of primary syphilis is based on the history, clinical features, and bacteriologic and serologic tests.

The differential diagnosis of oral chancre includes traumatic ulcer, aphthous ulcer, Behçet's disease, chancroid, tuberculous lesions, herpes simplex, infectious mononucleosis, and squamous cell carcinoma.

Laboratory tests include dark-field examination for T. pallidum. Serologic tests for syphilis must always be performed, but it should be remembered that, during the early primary phase, these tests may be negative.

Secondary Syphilis

The signs and symptoms of secondary syphilis begin 6 to 8 weeks after the appearance of the chancre, which may still be present at the time of initiation of this stage. The clinical features of secondary syphilis are classified in two major groups: constitutional symptoms and signs, which may precede or accompany mucocutaneous lesions and include malaise, low-grade fever, headache, lacrimation, sore throat, loss of appetite, weight loss, polyarthralgias and myalgias, generalized lymphadenopathy, which is a classic and constant finding along with splenomegaly. The enlarged lymph nodes are painless, discrete, mobile, and hard-rubbery on palpation; and generalized mucocutaneous manifestations, which include pruritus, nail involvement, macular, papular, pustular, nodular, follicular, and other lesions. Mucous membrane lesions are frequent and may appear alone or in association with skin lesions. The mucocutaneous lesions usually last 2 to 10 weeks and disappear without scarring.

Macular Syphilides

Macular syphilides (roseolas) are the earliest manifestations of secondary syphilis, remaining for a few days and usually are unnoticed. In the oral mucosa macular syphilides are most frequently found in the soft palate (Fig. **203**). Clinically, they appear as multiple red oval spots.

Mucous Patches

Mucous patches are by far the most frequent oral manifestation of secondary syphilis. They are flat or slightly raised, painless, oval or round papules with erosions or superficial ulcers covered by a grayish-white membrane. They are teeming with

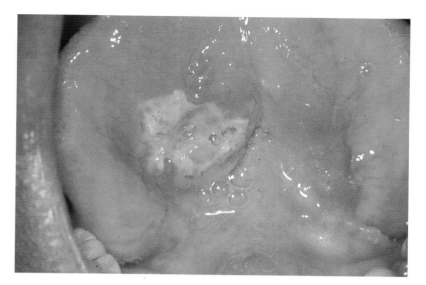

Fig. **201**. Solitary chancre on the ventral surface of the tongue.

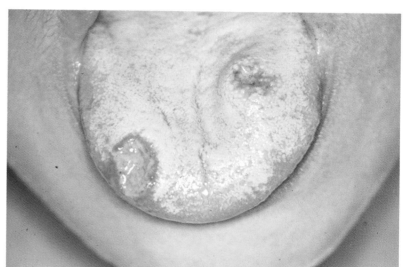

Fig. **202**. Two chancres on the tongue.

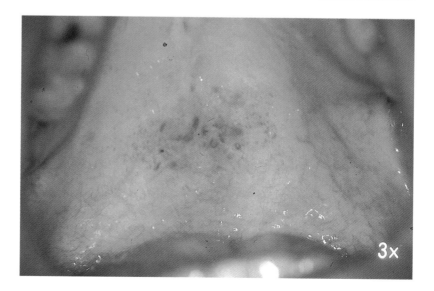

Fig. **203**. Macular syphilides on the soft palate.

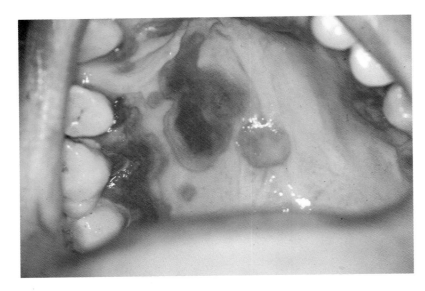

Fig. **204.** Mucous patches on the palate and gingiva.

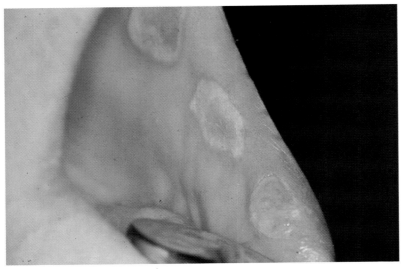

Fig. **205.** Mucous patches on the buccal and lip mucosa.

spirochetes and extremely contagious. The lesions may be surrounded by a red halo and vary in size from 3 to 10 mm or more in diameter. Mucous patches tend to arrange symmetrically, they are usually multiple and rarely occur as solitary lesions. They occur most frequently on the tongue, palate, tonsils, mucosal surface of the lips, commissures, buccal mucosa, gingiva, and the larynx (Figs. **204–206**). On occasion, mucous patches may be the only manifestation of secondary syphilis for a long period of time.

The differential diagnosis includes candidosis, lichen planus, leukoplakia, aphthous ulcers, herpetic gingivostomatitis, erythema multiforme, trauma, and infectious mononucleosis.

Laboratory test. Dark-field examination and immunofluorescence for the detection of T. pallidum may be a helpful diagnostic tool. In addition serologic tests (VDRL, RPR, FTA-ABS, TPI, TPHA) are positive.

Papular Syphilides

Papular syphilides are the most characteristic lesions of secondary syphilis and occur frequently on the skin (Fig. **207**) and rarely in the oral mucosa. The oral lesions usually coalesce, forming slightly raised, painless, firm, and round nodules with a grayish-white color (Fig. **208**). The lesions have a tendency to ulcerate and are usually located on the commissures and buccal mucosa and rarely in other areas. Papular syphilides and mucous patches are always associated with bilateral regional lymphadenopathy.

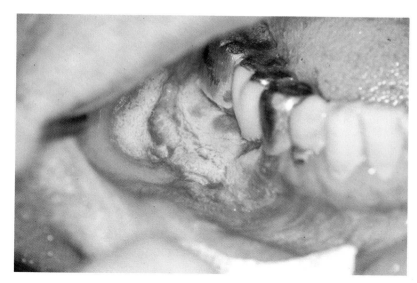

Fig. **206**. Mucous patches on the gingiva and alveolar mucosa.

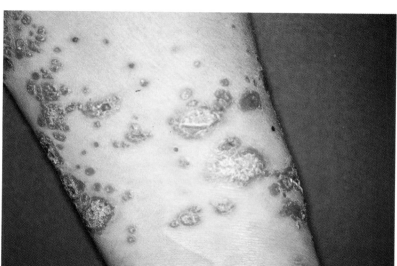

Fig. **207**. Papular syphilides on the skin.

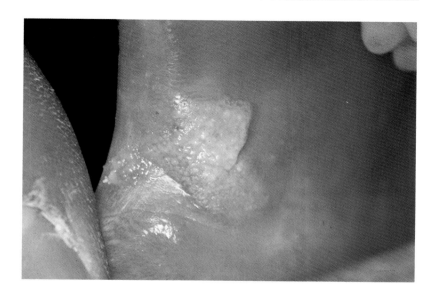

Fig. **208**. Papular syphilides on the buccal mucosa.

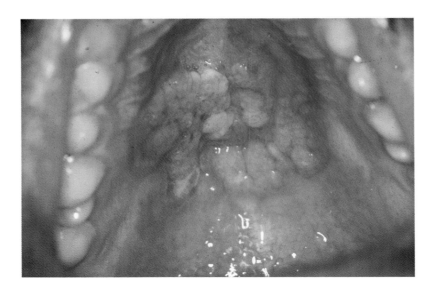

Fig. **209**. Condylomata lata on the palate.

Condylomata Lata

In moistened skin areas, the eroded papular syphilides have the tendency to coalesce and to hypertrophy, forming elevated, vegetating, or papillomatous lesions, the condylomata lata. The most frequent localizations of condylomata lata are the perigenital-perianal area, axillae, submammary, and umbilical areas. Condylomata lata rarely appear in the oral cavity, usually at the corners of the mouth and the palate (Fig. **209**). They are painless, slightly exophytic, multiple lesions with an irregular surface and are contagious.

Late Syphilis

After a latency period of 4 to 7 years or more, severe clinical manifestations of late syphilis may develop. The main manifestations of late syphilis are mucocutaneous lesions, cardiovascular lesions, and neurosyphilis. Late syphilis is now rare in many western countries. The oral lesions of late syphilis include gummas, atrophic glossitis, and interstitial glossitis.

Gumma

Gumma is a syphilitic granulomatous lesion that originates as a subcutaneous mass secondarily extending both to the epithelium and the deeper tissues. Gumma appears initially as a painless elastic tumor that has a tendency to necrose, forming a characteristic stringy mass. A punched-out ulcer forms and finally heals, leaving a scar. The size varies from 1 to 10 cm. The sites of predilection are the legs, scalp, face, and chest. Gummas are frequently located on the hard palate, which they may destroy and perforate (Fig. **210**). They may also involve the soft palate and rarely other oral regions.

The differential diagnosis includes carcinoma or other malignant tumors, leprosy, lethal midline granuloma, lymphoma.

Atrophic Glossitis

The tongue is frequently involved in late syphilis. Clinically, there is atrophy of the filiform and fungiform papillae, and the dorsum becomes smooth and atrophic. Vasculitis finally ending in an obliterative endarteritis is the process underlying these changes.

Atrophic syphilitic glossitis may lead to the development of leukoplakia and squamous cell carcinoma (Fig. **211**).

The differential diagnosis includes atrophic lichen planus and Plummer-Vinson syndrome.

Interstitial Glossitis

Late syphilis of the tongue may occur either as a solitary gumma or most common as a diffuse gummatous infiltration, which heals spontaneously, leading to interstitial glossitis. This is the result of contracture of the lingual musculature after the healing of gummas. The tongue appears smoothly lobulated with irregular deep fissures (Fig. **212**).

Leukoplakia and squamous cell carcinoma may develop.

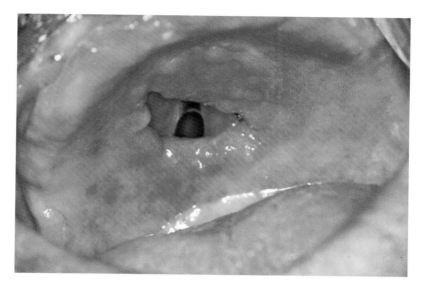

Fig. **210**. Gumma, perforation of the hard palate.

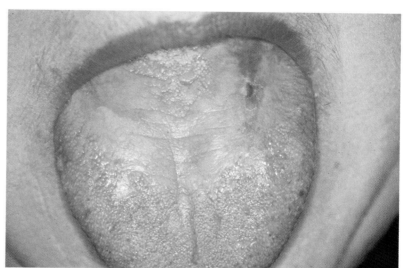

Fig. **211**. Atrophic glossitis in late syphilis.

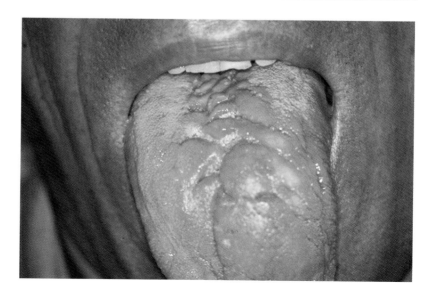

Fig. **212**. Interstitial glossitis in late syphilis.

Treatment. Penicillin is the treatment for all stages of syphilis. The schedules and dosages are internationally established and depend on the stage of the disease. If penicillin allergy exists, erythromycin or cephalosporins may be administered.

Congenital Syphilis

Congenital (prenatal) syphilis is transmitted by the mother to the fetus in utero. It is classified as early if the disease manifests before age 2 years, late if it becomes apparent after age 2 years and stigmata, which are developmental changes without active infection.

The most common stigmata are high arched palate, short mandible, rhagades at the commissures, saddle nose, frontal bossing, Hutchinson's teeth, and dysplastic molars.

The dysplastic permanent incisors comprise, along with interstitial keratitis and eighth nerve deafness, the classic Hutchinson's triad, and they are the most common findings of congenital syphilis. Clinically, the upper central permanent incisors are widely spaced and shorter than the lateral incisors. They are conical or barrel-shaped and at the biting surfaces are usually smaller than at the gingival margins (Fig. 213). Notched biting surfaces may be present as a result of defective enamel. Similar changes may exist in the lateral incisors (although to a lesser degree), and the teeth may be irregularly spaced. The permanent first molars may be dysplastic (Moon's molars, Fournier's molars, mulberry molars). Usually the first lower molars are affected. Affected teeth are narrower on their occlusal surfaces and have supernumerary cusps.

Chancroid

Chancroid is an acute venereal disease caused by Hemophilus ducreyi a gram-negative bacillus. The disease is rare in Europe and the United States and occurs most frequently in underdeveloped countries, especially in communities with poor hygiene. The disease is usually sexually transmitted. Genital and perianal regions are most commonly affected. Oral lesions, which occur after orogenital contact, are extremely rare. After an incubation period of 2 to 5 days, the disease begins as a small red papule or macule that soon becomes pustular and finally ulcerates. The lesions of chancroid are not pathognomonic. The ulcer is round or oval, 1 mm to 2 cm in diameter with slightly raised border and a soft base (Fig. 214). It is covered with a gray-whitish exudate and is surrounded by a red halo. It is painful and usually accompanied by bilateral or unilateral lymphadenopathy.

The differential diagnosis includes aphthous ulcer, traumatic ulcer, primary and secondary syphilis.

Laboratory tests that are helpful in establishing the diagnosis include bacteriologic stains of smears and culture.

Treatment. Erythromycin is the drug of choice. In addition, the combination of sulfamethoxazole and trimethoprim or other antibiotics are effective.

Gonococcal Stomatitis

Gonorrhea is a common venereal disease caused by the gram-negative diplococcus **Neisseria gonorrhoeae.** It occurs at all ages and affects both sexes. Gonorrhea is sexually transmitted and involves the genitals, the anal canal, the pharynx, and rarely the oral cavity. Gonococcal stomatitis and pharyngitis are the result of fellatio and are more common in prostitutes and homosexual men. Gonococcal stomatitis is rare without specific clinical signs. The oral mucosa is red, inflamed, and the patient complains of itching and burning. Rarely, erosions and ulcers covered with a whitish pseudomembrane may occur (Fig. 215).

Gonococcal pharyngitis is more frequent and can be manifested as a sore throat or as a diffuse or patchy erythema and edema with or without tiny pustules of the tonsillar pillars and uvula. Notably, oral gonococcal infection may be asymptomatic.

The differential diagnosis includes streptococcal stomatitis, herpetic infection, and candidosis.

Laboratory identification of the organisms by Gram's stain or culture establish definitive diagnosis.

Treatment. Oral lesions are self-limited and colonization disappears within 3 months. Penicillin, tetracycline, amoxicillin, and ampicillin in different regimens may eradicate the disease.

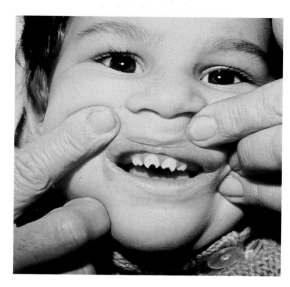

Fig. **213**. Congenital syphilis, Hutchinson's teeth.

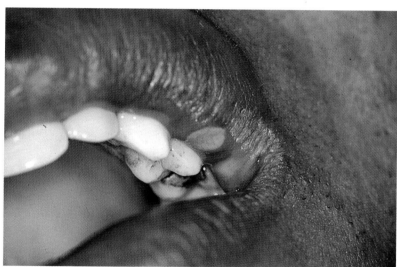

Fig. **214**. Chancroid, round ulcer on the upper lip.

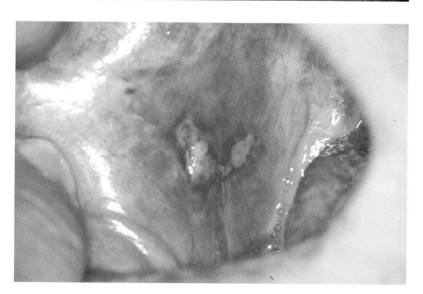

Fig. **215**. Gonococcal stomatitis, erythema and erosions on the buccal mucosa.

Tuberculosis

The oral mucosa is a rare location of tuberculous infection. The oral infection is usually secondary to pulmonary tuberculosis. The most common secondary lesion of the oral mucosa is the tuberculous ulcer. Clinically, the ulcer is painless, irregular with a thin undermined border. The surface of the ulcer is vegetating and usually covered by a gray-yellowish exudate. The surrounding tissue is mildly indurated, with inflammation. The size varies from 1 to 5 cm. The dorsal surface of the tongue is most commonly affected, followed by the palate, buccal mucosa, and lips (Figs. **216, 217**). Rarely, a tuberculous ulcer of the oral cavity may be the only manifestation of an otherwise silent tuberculosis. Tuberculous osteomyelitis of the jaws and periapical tuberculous granuloma may also occur. Regional lymphadenopathy usually accompanies the oral lesions. Tuberculosis of cervical lymph nodes may lead to scrofula, with breakdown of the skin overlying the infected lymph nodes and multiple fistula formation (Fig. **218**).

The differential diagnosis includes squamous cell carcinoma, syphilis, lymphoma, major aphthous ulcer, traumatic ulcer, Wegener's granulomatosis, lethal midline granuloma, and eosinophilic ulcer.

Laboratory tests for the diagnosis of tuberculosis are histopathologic examination, cultures, and a tuberculin skin test. Chest radiographs frequently reveal pulmonary tuberculosis.

Treatment. Therapy consists of systemic anti-tuberculous drugs and is best to be left to the specialist physician.

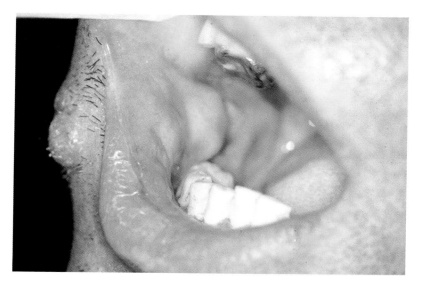

Fig. **222**. Actinomycosis, nodules and sinus of the buccal mucosa.

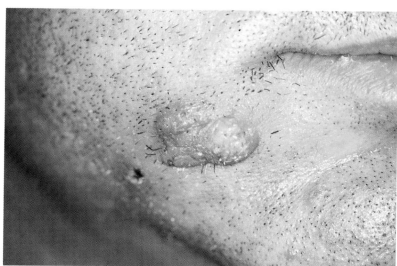

Fig. **223**. Actinomycosis, multiple nodules and sinus of the skin.

17. Fungal Infections

Candidosis

Candidosis is the most frequent fungal infection and is caused by Candida albicans, a fungus that is part of the normal oral flora in up to 50% of persons. Predisposing factors of oral candidosis include local factors, diabetes mellitus, iron deficiency anemia, chronic diseases, malignancies, antibiotics, corticosteroid and other immunosuppressive drugs, radiation, hypoparathyroidism, Addison's disease, and humoral and cell-mediated immunodeficiency. In addition, oral candidosis is an early opportunistic infection that occurs in about two-thirds of the patients with or at high risk for the acquired immune deficiency syndrome (AIDS). Newborns and infants are also particularly susceptible to candidosis. Oral candidosis has a broad spectrum of clinical manifestations. However, a satisfactory classification includes the following clinical varieties.

Acute Pseudomembranous Candidosis (Thrush)

Thrush is the most common form of the disease and is clinically characterized by creamy white or whitish yellow, slightly elevated spots or plaques, which can be easily detached, leaving a raw underlying reddish or normal surface. These lesions may be localized or generalized and may appear at any oral site, but more frequently on the buccal mucosa, the tongue, and the soft and hard palate (Fig. 224, 225). Subjective complaints include xerostomia and slight burning sensation. This form of candidosis is common in human immunodeficiency virus (HIV) infection.

Acute Atrophic Candidosis

Acute atrophic candidosis is usually observed in patients receiving broad-spectrum antibiotics, corticosteroids, or other immunosuppressive agents. Clinically, there are erythematous areas with very few whitish lesions and have a predilection for the dorsal surface of the tongue (Fig. 226). Acute atrophic candidosis frequently causes intense burning and may be associated with HIV infection.

Chronic Atrophic Candidosis

Chronic atrophic candidosis is synonymous with the term "denture stomatitis or denture sore mouth." It is a common form of oral candidosis among denture wearers. Clinically, chronic atrophic candidosis is characterized by a diffuse erythema and slight edema of the palatal mucosa underneath the denture. Scattered white spots or plaques may occasionally be seen. Angular cheilitis is often associated with this form of candidosis (Fig. 227).

Chronic Hyperplastic Candidosis, or Candidal Leukoplakia

Chronic hyperplastic candidosis is a chronic form of candidosis that is characterized by deep infiltration of the oral tissues by fungal hyphae. Clinically, it is characterized by white, firm, and raised plaques occasionally surrounded by erythema (Fig. 228). The lesions may persist for years, do not detach, and usually are located on the dorsum of the tongue, the buccal mucosa, and rarely in other areas. Rarely, lesions of this form of candidosis have been seen in patients with HIV infection. It has been suggested that chronic hyperplastic candidosis predisposes to squamous cell carcinoma and is therefore a precancerous lesion.

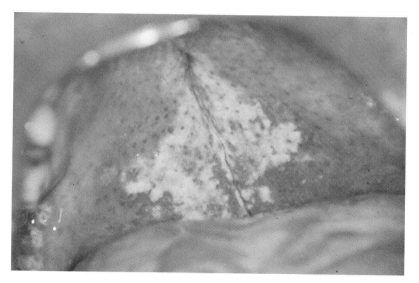

Fig. **224**. Acute pseudomembranous candidosis.

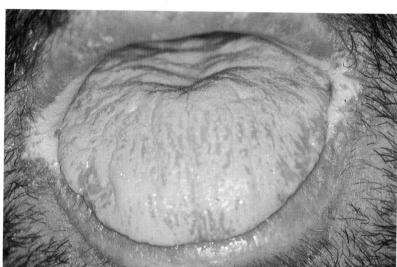

Fig. **225**. Acute pseudomembranous candidosis.

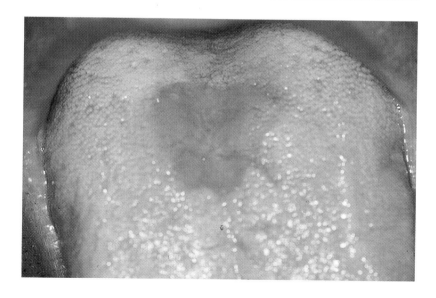

Fig. **226**. Acute atrophic candidosis.

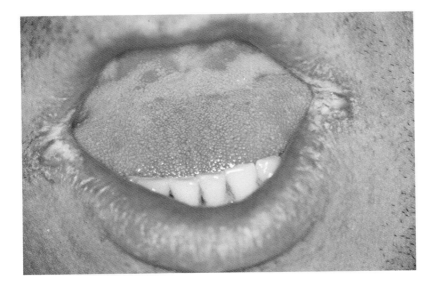

Fig. **227**. Chronic atrophic candidosis.

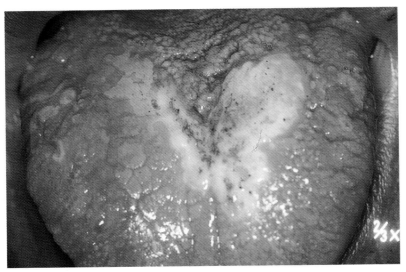

Fig. **228**. Chronic hyperplastic candidosis.

Chronic Multifocal Candidosis

Chronic multifocal candidosis is a rare form that is characterized by white, adherent, firm plaques on a reddish base. Sometimes, these lesions may form small nodules or have a verrucous surface. The lesions are usually multiple and are located on the buccal mucosa, the retrocommissural area, the palate, the dorsum of the tongue, and last for a long period (Figs. **229, 230**).

Papillary Hyperplasia of the Palate

Papillary hyperplasia of the palate is a rare chronic form of candidosis that usually affects persons with a high arched palate who do not wear dentures. Clinically, multiple small spherical nodules appear on the palate, which is usually red (Fig. **231**). This lesion should not be confused with denture stomatitis, which appears in persons wearing dentures.

19. Diseases with Possible Immunopathogenesis

Recurrent Aphthous Ulcers

Recurrent aphthous ulcers are the most common lesions of the oral mucosa and affect 10 to 30% of the population. The exact cause remains unknown, although numerous possible etiologic factors have been suggested, such as iron, vitamin B_{12} or folic acid deficiency, and viral or bacterial infection, especially with Streptococcus species (S. sanguis, S. mitis).

Trauma, endocrine disturbances, emotional stress, and allergy are considered the most important predisposing factors. In women the lesions may occur in a cyclic pattern a few days before menstruation. Recent evidence supports the concept that cell-mediated and humoral immunity to oral mucosal antigens play a primary role in the pathogenesis of recurrent aphthous ulcers and Behçet's syndrome. Recurrent aphthous ulcers have been classified into four varieties based on clinical criteria: minor, major, herpetiform ulcers, and aphthae associated with Behçet's syndrome.

Minor Aphthous Ulcers

Minor aphthous ulcers are the most common form of the disease. They occur somewhat more frequently in females than in males during the second and third decades, although they may appear at any age. A prodromal burning sensation 24 to 48 hours before the appearance of the ulcer is recognized. Clinically, the ulcers are small, 2 to 6 mm in diameter, oval, and very painful, covered by a yellow-white membrane that represents necrotic tissue (Fig. 241). They are well circumscribed and surrounded by a thin erythematous halo. A vesicular stage does not exist.

Ulcers can be single or multiple (2 to 6), they generally persist 5 to 8 days, and gradually heal with no evidence of scarring. They recur usually at 1- to 5-month intervals. The most common sites of occurrence are the nonkeratinized (movable) oral mucosa (buccal mucosa, lips, tongue, mucolabial and mucobuccal folds). The lesions are extremely rare on the hard palate and gingiva.

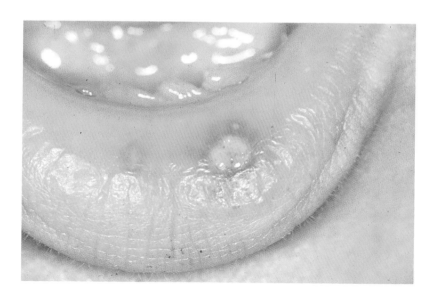

Fig. 241. Minor aphthous ulcer.

Major Aphthous Ulcers

Major aphthous ulcers are currently believed to be a more severe form of aphthous ulcerations. They were previously thought to represent a separate disease entity known as periadenitis mucosa necrotica recurrens, or Sutton's disease. These ulcers are usually one to five in number and 1 to 2 cm in diameter each, deep and extremely painful (Figs. **242, 243**). The most common sites of occurrence are the lips, buccal mucosa, tongue, and soft palate. They may persist for 3 to 6 weeks, leave a scar on healing in cases of very deep ulcers, and recur, often at 1- to 3-month intervals.

The diagnosis of minor and major aphthous ulcers is based exclusively on clinical criteria. In addition, HLA-B12, A2, AW29, and DR7 antigens are found with slightly increased frequency in patients with aphthous ulcers.

The differential diagnosis of minor and major aphthous ulcers should include herpes simplex, hand-foot-and-mouth disease, syphilitic chancre and mucous patches of secondary syphilis, cyclic neutropenia, erythema multiforme, less frequently stomatitis venenata and medicamentosa, and rarely malignant ulcers.

Treatment. Topical application of a steroid ointment reduces discomfort and decreases the duration of the lesions. Topical anesthetics, antibiotics, mouthwashes, cauterizing chemicals, etc., have been used. In severe cases, intralesional steroid injection or systemic steroids in a low dose (10 to 20 mg prednisone) for 5 to 10 days reduce the pain dramatically.

Herpetiform Ulcers

Herpetiform ulcers, or herpetiform stomatitis, was first described by Cook in 1960, who pointed out the clinical similarities of this disease to the lesions of herpes simplex and the corresponding histologic, microbiologic, and immunologic differences. The disease presents as multiple (10 to 100 in number) small shallow ulcers, 1 to 2 mm in diameter, with a thin red halo, which gradually coalesce to larger irregular lesions (Fig. **244**). The lesions are very painful and may occur at any site of the oral mucosa, where they persist for 1 to 2 weeks and recur often over a period of 1 to 3 years.

The most common age of onset is between 20 and 30 years. Although the exact nature of the disease is unknown, it is considered appropriate to include it as a variant of recurrent aphthous ulcers.

The differential diagnosis includes primary herpetic gingivostomatitis, herpangina, and erythema multiforme.

Treatment is symptomatic. Low doses of corticosteroids (15 to 20 mg prednisone) for 3 to 5 days may be useful in severe cases.

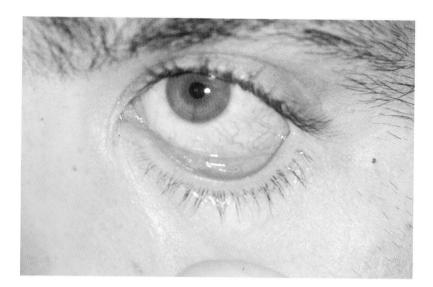

Fig. **251**. Reiter's syndrome, conjunctivitis.

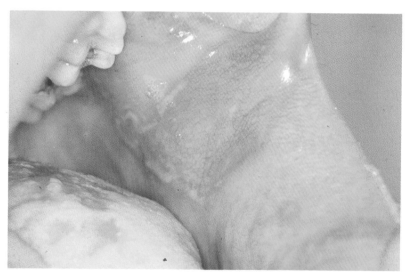

Fig. **252**. Reiter's syndrome, red areas surrounded by whitish annular lines on the buccal mucosa.

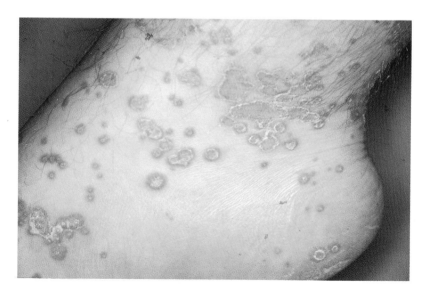

Fig. **253**. Reiter's syndrome, psoriasiform lesions on the skin.

onset of the disease, they may be important for the diagnosis. Asymmetrical arthritis of the large joints is the most important and early manifestation and occasionally may produce disability. Cardiovascular and neurologic disorders and amyloidosis may rarely occur.

The differential diagnosis of the oral lesions includes erythema multiforme, Stevens-Johnson syndrome, psoriasis, Behçet's syndrome, geographic tongue and stomatitis.

Laboratory tests. There is no accurate test. However, histopathologic and radiographic examinations are helpful.

Treatment. It is nonspecific and symptomatic. Nonsteroidal anti-inflammatory drugs, salicylates, and tetracyclines may be helpful.

Wegener's Granulomatosis

Wegener's granulomatosis is a rare chronic granulomatous disease of unknown cause, although an immunologic mechanism is probably related to the pathogenesis. The disease is characterized by necrotizing granulomatous lesions of the upper and lower respiratory tract, generalized focal necrotizing vasculitis involving both veins and arteries, and necrotizing glomerulitis that may progress to granulomatous glomerulonephritis. Oral lesions in Wegener's granulomatosis are fairly common, although the true incidence is not known. Clinically, the lesions appear as solitary or multiple ulcers surrounded by an inflammatory zone (Fig. **254**). The tongue, palate, and buccal mucosa are commonly affected. Rarely, a peculiar gingival enlargement may be an early feature of the disease. The gingiva is enlarged with a red, papillary granulomatous surface. Skin lesions occur in half of the patients and are characterized by papules, petechiae, plaques, and ulcers. Ocular, cardiac, joint, and neurologic manifestations may also occur. The pulmonary and renal involvement are the most common and severe manifestations of the disease. The prognosis is usually unfavorable, although recently limited forms of the disease with a better course have been described.

The differential diagnosis includes lethal midline granuloma, tuberculous ulcers, squamous cell carcinoma, leukemia, and lymphoma.

Laboratory tests that are helpful in establishing the diagnosis include histopathologic examination, chest radiographs, blood count, and urinalysis.

Treatment. A combined therapy with steroids, cyclophosphamide, and azathioprine have improved the prognosis of the disease.

Lethal Midline Granuloma

Lethal midline granuloma represents a disease spectrum characterized by progressive unrelenting ulceration and necrosis involving the nasal cavity, palate, and the midline segment of the face. The precise pathogenesis remains unknown. Many investigators consider that lethal midline granuloma and Wegener's granulomatosis are extremes of a spectrum. However, recent evidence disputes this view, and under the term "lethal midline granuloma" three varieties may be included: the "essentially inflammatory," or idiopathic midline granuloma; the "obviously neoplastic," or polymorphic reticulosis, which is a lymphoproliferative disorder; and a lymphoma with low-grade malignancy. Clinically, the disease is characterized by prodromal signs and symptoms, such as epistaxis, slight pain, nasal stuffiness, foul-smelling secretions, and nasal obstruction with a purulent discharge. Nonhealing ulceration and necrosis of the palate, alveolar processes, retromolar pad, and the nasal cavity occur frequently (Fig. **255**). These lesions deteriorate rather rapidly, causing destruction and perforation of the palate, nasal septum and bones, and the neighboring bony structures, resulting in severe disfiguration. The prognosis is unfavorable, with an extremely high fatality rate.

The differential diagnosis includes Wegener's granulomatosis, leprosy, syphilitic gumma, lymphoma, squamous cell carcinoma, tuberculosis, necrotizing sialometaplasia, and deep mycotic infections.

Laboratory test. Histopathologic examination is helpful in establishing the diagnosis.

Treatment. Radiation has been reported to have therapeutic value. Steroids and other cytotoxic agents have failed to change the prognosis.

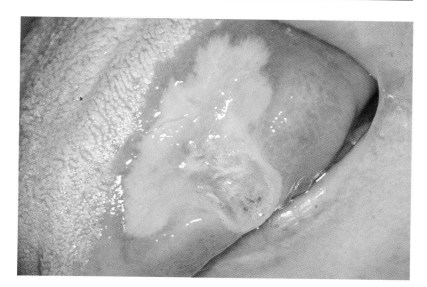

Fig. **254**. Wegener's granulomatosis, large ulcer surrounded by an erythematous zone on the tongue.

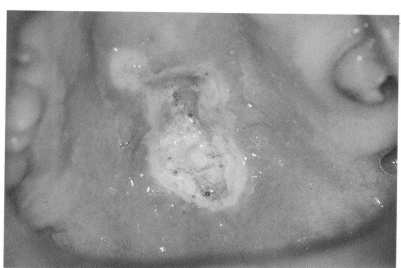

Fig. **255**. Lethal midline granuloma, nonhealing ulcer and necrosis on the palate.

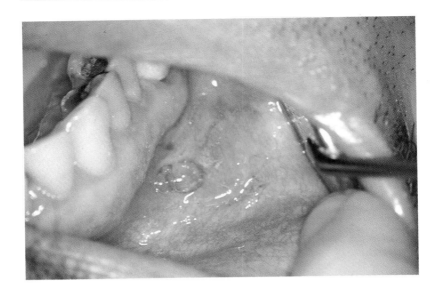

Fig. **256**. Crohn's disease, granulomatous lesion on the mucobuccal groove.

Crohn's Disease

Crohn's disease, or regional enteritis, is a chronic inflammatory disease involving the ileum and other parts of the gastrointestinal tract. The cause remains obscure, although an immune mechanism probably participates in the pathogenesis. The disease usually affects young persons between 20 and 30 years of age, and clinically presents with abdominal pain, diarrhea, weight loss, vomiting, low-grade fever, and rectal bleeding. Extra-abdominal manifestations of the disease include spondylitis, arthritis, uveitis, and oral manifestations. Oral lesions have been found in 10 to 20% of patients with Crohn's disease, and they may either precede or follow the intestinal involvement. Clinically, the most frequently affected areas are the buccal mucosa and the mucobuccal fold, where the changes appear as edematous, hypertrophic, or granulomatous lesions with or without ulcers (Fig. **256**). Diffuse raised nodules resulting in a "cobblestone" appearance of the buccal mucosa or epulis fissuratum-like lesions may also occur. Granulomatous lip swelling, angular cheilitis, diffuse granular erythematous gingival swelling, and palatal ulceration may be seen. In addition, nonspecific aphthous-like lesions are frequently associated with Crohn's disease. The oral lesions usually regress when intestinal symptoms are in remission.

The differential diagnosis includes pyogenic granuloma, epulis fissuratum, tuberculosis, sarcoidosis, cheilitis granulomatosa, and Melkersson-Rosenthal syndrome.

Laboratory test. Histopathologic examination and radiologic studies of the bowel are helpful in establishing the diagnosis.

Treatment. Topical corticosteroids; systemic corticosteroids, sulfonamides, and immunosuppressive agents in severe cases.

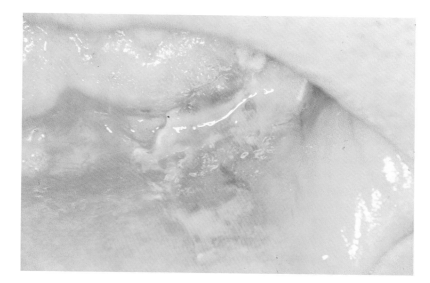

Fig. **281**. Pemphigus foliaceus, erosions on the mucolabial groove and lip mucosa.

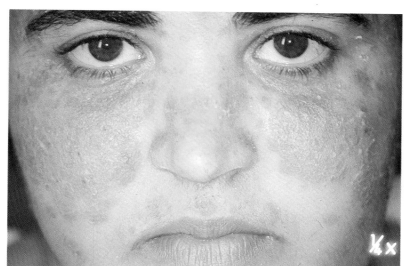

Fig. **282**. Pemphigus erythematosus, characteristic erythema and superficial crusting lesions on the "butterfly" area of the face.

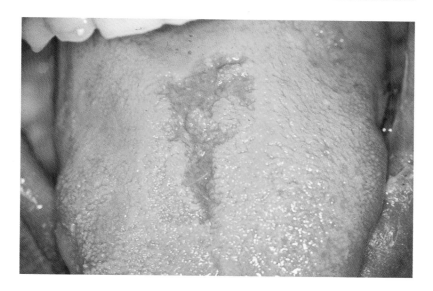

Fig. **283**. Pemphigus erythematosus, localized erosion on the dorsum of the tongue.

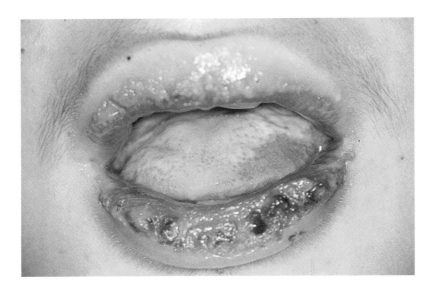

Fig. **284**. Juvenile pemphigus vulgaris, severe erosions on the lips.

Juvenile Pemphigus Vulgaris

Pemphigus very rarely affects persons less than 20 years of age. It is now well documented that pemphigus vulgaris, foliaceus, and erythematosus occur in children, too, but the oral mucosa is usually affected by pemphigus vulgaris. It has been reported that in 13 of 14 young patients with pemphigus vulgaris (93%) the disease began in the oral cavity and the female to male ratio was 1.8:1. Clinically localized or widespread superficial erosions are seen, which may persist and exhibit a tendency to enlarge (Fig. **284**). The clinical and laboratory features of juvenile pemphigus are similar to those seen in pemphigus of the adults.

The differential diagnosis includes other bullous diseases affecting children, such as herpetic gingivostomatitis, juvenile bullous pemphigoid, juvenile dermatitis herpetiformis, erythema multiforme, cicatricial pemphigoid of childhood, linear immunoglobulin A (IgA) disease of childhood.

Cicatricial Pemphigoid

Cicatricial pemphigoid, or benign mucous membrane pemphigoid, is a chronic bullous disease of autoimmune origin that preferentially affects mucous membranes and results in atrophy of the epithelium and sometimes in scarring. The disease occurs more frequently in women than in men (1.5:1), with a mean age of onset of 66 years. The oral mucosa is invariably affected and, in 95% of the cases, the mouth is the initial site of involvement. The most consistent oral lesions are those involving the gingiva, although ultimately other sites in the oral cavity may be involved. The mucosal lesions are recurrent vesicles or small bullae that rupture, leaving a raw eroded surface that finally heals by scar formation (Fig. **285**). Oral lesions are usually localized, and rarely widespread involvement is seen (Fig. **286**). Frequently, the disease affects exclusively the gingiva in the form of desquamative gingivitis (Fig. **287**). The ocular lesions consist of conjunctivitis, symblepharon, trichiasis, dryness, and opacity of the cornea frequently leading to complete blindness (Figs. **288, 289**). Less commonly, other mucosae (genitals, anus, nose, pharynx, esophagus, larynx) are involved (Fig. **290**). Skin lesions occur in about 10 to 20% of the cases and consist of bullae that usually appear on the scalp, face, and neck and may heal with or without scarring.

The differential diagnosis includes pemphigus vulgaris, bullous pemphigoid, bullous and erosive lichen planus, dermatitis herpetiformis, erythema multiforme, Stevens-Johnson syndrome, and lupus erythematosus.

Laboratory tests. Helpful laboratory tests include histopathologic examination and direct immunofluorescence of oral mucosa biopsy specimens.

Treatment. Systemic steroid and immunosuppressive drugs. In mild cases topical steroids (cream or intralesional injection) may be useful.

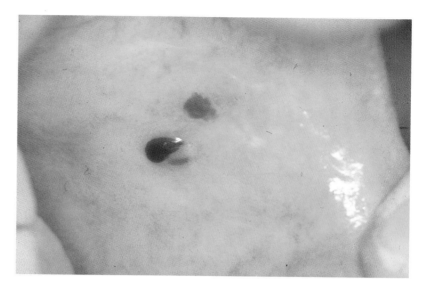

Fig. **285**. Cicatricial pemphigoid, intact hemorrhagic bullae on the buccal mucosa.

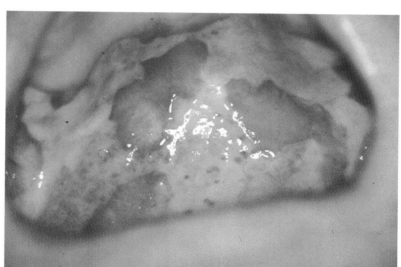

Fig. **286**. Cicatricial pemphigoid, severe erosions on the palate.

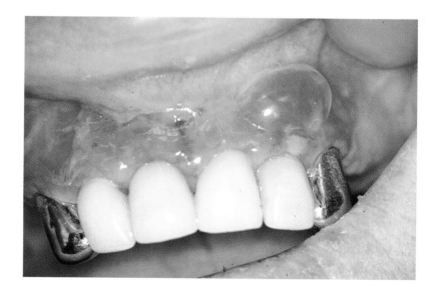

Fig. **287**. Cicatricial pemphigoid, presenting as desquamative gingivitis.

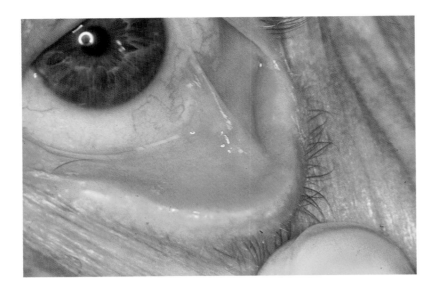

Fig. **288**. Cicatricial pemphigoid, conjunctivitis and symblepharon.

Cicatricial Pemphigoid of Childhood

Cicatricial pemphigoid is a chronic autoimmune bullous disease that affects almost exclusively middle-aged and elderly persons. However, at least seven well-documented cases of cicatricial pemphigoid of childhood have been recorded so far. Five of the patients were girls and two were boys, age 4 to 18 years. All patients except one had oral lesions, and in three, desquamative gingivitis was the cardinal manifestation of the disease (Fig. **291**). The clinical manifestations of oral mucosa, eyes, genitalia, anus, and skin are identical to those seen in cicatricial pemphigoid of adulthood.

The differential diagnosis includes juvenile bullous pemphigoid, juvenile pemphigus, dermatitis herpetiformis of childhood, childhood cicatricial pemphigoid with linear IgA deposits, chronic bullous disease of childhood, and epidermolysis bullosa.

Laboratory tests. Histopathologic examination, direct and indirect immunofluorescent tests confirm the diagnosis.

Treatment. Corticosteroids topically or systemically.

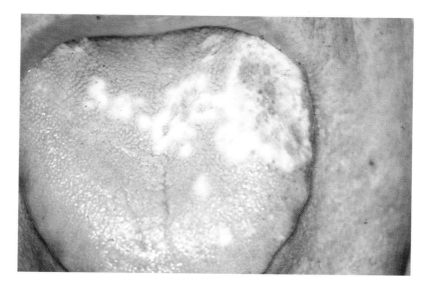

Fig. **299**. Lichen planus, reticular form, of the tongue.

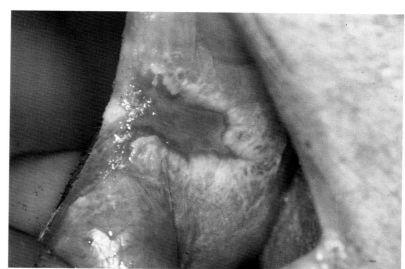

Fig. **300**. Lichen planus, erosive form, of the buccal mucosa.

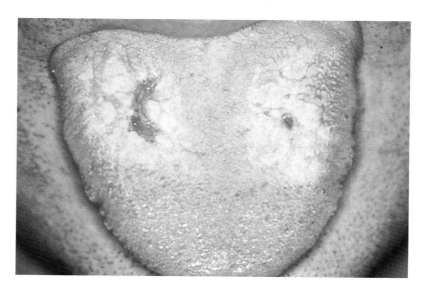

Fig. **301**. Lichen planus, erosive and hypertrophic form, of the tongue.

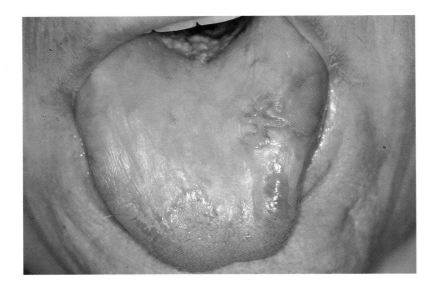

Fig. **302**. Lichen planus, atrophic form, of the dorsum of the tongue.

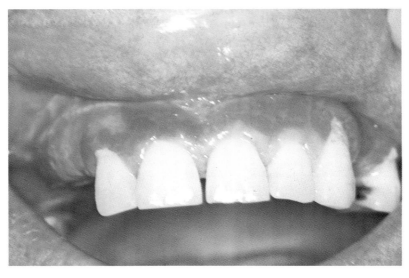

Fig. **303**. Lichen planus, presenting as desquamative gingivitis.

giva, and rarely the lips, palate, and floor of the mouth. The lesions are usually symmetrical and asymptomatic or cause mild discomfort, such as a burning sensation, irritation after contact with certain foods, and an unpleasant feeling of roughness in the mouth. However, erosive and bullous forms tend to be painful. The prognosis is good, although it has been suggested that there is a possibility of malignant transformation in the erosive and atrophic forms.

The differential diagnosis includes lupus erythematosus, erythroplakia, erythema multiforme, cicatricial pemphigoid, bullous pemphigoid, pemphigus, dermatitis herpetiformis, secondary syphilis and syphilitic glossitis, candidosis, and leukoplakia.

Laboratory tests. Histopathologic examination and direct immunofluorescent examinations help in establishing the diagnosis.

Treatment. No therapy is needed when the lesions are asymptomatic. In the erosive form of lichen planus topical, injectable, or systemic steroids are helpful. Aromatic retinoids (etretinate) have also been used with partial success.

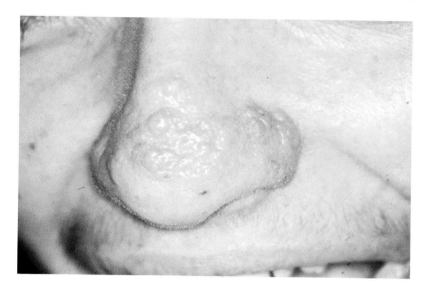

Fig. **330**. Lipoid proteinosis, nodules on the nose.

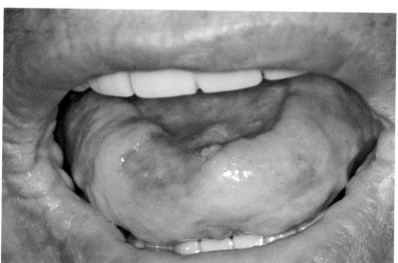

Fig. **331**. Lipoid proteinosis, large and glossy tongue.

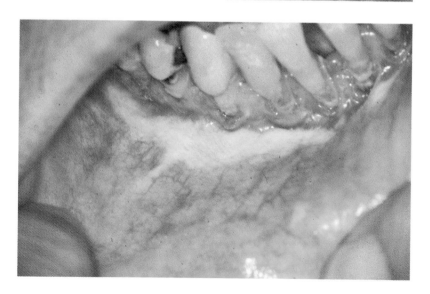

Fig. **332**. Xanthomas of the muco-labial fold mucosa.

The differential diagnosis includes leukoplakia, Fordyce's granules, verruciform xanthoma, and focal epithelial hyperplasia.

Laboratory tests to confirm the diagnosis are histopathologic examination and serologic determination of lipids.

Treatment. There is no topical treatment.

Porphyrias

Porphyrias are a rare group of disorders characterized by a defect in porphyrin metabolism, resulting in overproduction of porphyrins and their precursors. Each type is characterized by a deficient activity of specific enzymes in heme synthesis and abnormal porphyrin patterns found either in the urine, feces, or in different tissues. On the basis of the tissue origin of abnormal porphyrin synthesis, the human porphyrias are classified into three major groups with several types: erythropoietic (congenital erythropoietic porphyria, erythropoietic coproporphyria), hepatic (acute intermittent porphyria, variegate porphyria, Chester porphyria, porphyria cutanea tarda, hereditary coproporphyria), and erythrohepatic (erythrohepatic protoporphyria, hepatoerythropoietic porphyria). Photosensitivity of the skin is seen in almost all types of porphyria. In addition, skin fragility, erythema, vesicles, bullae, erosions, hyperpigmentation, hypertrichosis, scars, scarring alopecia, milia, etc., are common findings. Light-exposed areas of the skin are primarily affected, along with systemic signs and symptoms.

Congenital porphyria (Günther's disease) is a rare genetic type characterized by severe cutaneous lesions, hemolytic anemia, and splenomegaly. The presence of red-brown teeth due to incorporation of porphyrins into the developing teeth is an important diagnostic finding in both deciduous and permanent dentition. Under ultraviolet light, the teeth exhibit a characteristic reddish pink fluorescence. The oral mucosa is rarely affected in porphyrias. However, erythema, vesicles, bullae, ulcers, atrophy but no scarring may appear in congenital erythropoietic porphyria and occasionally in porphyria cutanea tarda. The oral lesions usually develop on the vermilion border of the lips, commissures, labial mucosa, anterior vestibular alveolar mucosa, and gingiva (Figs. **333, 334**).

The differential diagnosis includes epidermolysis bullosa, chronic bullous diseases, lipoid proteinosis, pellagra, and drug-induced photosensitivity.

Laboratory tests to establish the diagnosis are biochemical tests, histopathologic examination, and direct immunofluorescence.

Treatment is best left to the specialist.

Hemochromatosis

Hemochromatosis is a rare inherited metabolic disorder of unknown cause resulting in deposition of large amounts of iron in the internal organs. Clinically, the disorder is characterized by the coexistence of diabetes mellitus, liver cirrhosis, hyperpigmentation, and less frequently gonadal deficiency, cardiac failure, and joint disorders. Hyperpigmentation may appear both in skin and mucous membranes (oral and conjunctiva). The skin acquires a generalized gray-brown pigmentation in almost all cases. The oral mucosa shows diffuse homogeneous pigmentation of gray-brown or deep brown hue in about 20% of the cases. The buccal mucosa and the attached gingiva are the most frequently involved sites (Fig. **335**). In addition, major and minor salivary gland involvement has been reported.

The differential diagnosis includes Addison's disease, drug-induced hyperpigmentation, and normal pigmentation in dark-skinned persons.

Laboratory tests. Routine laboratory tests may reveal evidence of diabetes mellitus and liver dysfunction. In addition, the serum determination of iron, transferrin, and ferritin are helpful in establishing the diagnosis according to standard criteria.

Treatment is best left to the specialist.

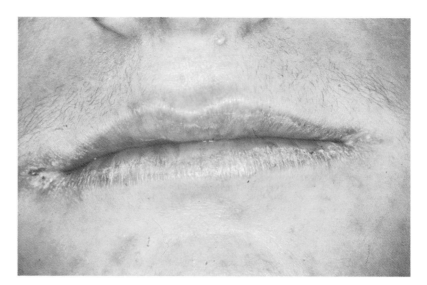

Fig. **333**. Porphyria cutanea tarda, erythema of the lips and angular cheilitis.

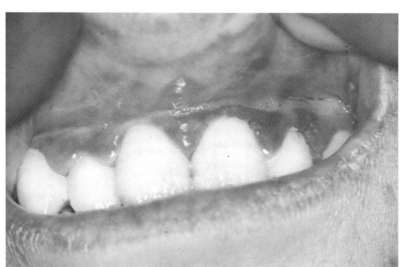

Fig. **334**. Porphyria cutanea tarda, diffuse erythema on the gingiva and upper lip mucosa.

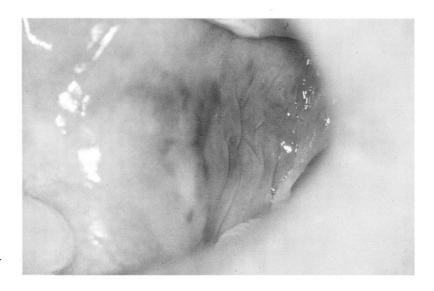

Fig. **335**. Hemochromatosis, pigmentation of the buccal mucosa.

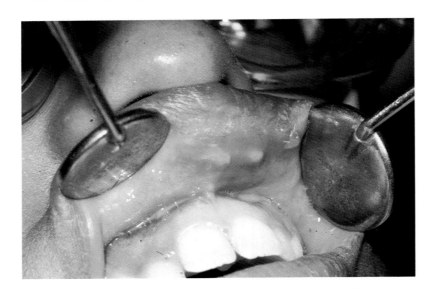

Fig. **336**. Cystic fibrosis, localized swelling of the upper lip.

Cystic Fibrosis

Cystic fibrosis, or mucoviscidosis, is a genetic disease transmitted as an autosomal recessive trait. The exact biochemical defect is unknown. The disease is characterized by dysfunction of the exocrine glands, particularly the exocrine pancreas, bronchial, tracheal, and gastrointestinal tract glands. The cardinal manifestations are chronic pulmonary infections, pancreatic insufficiency, cirrhosis, and skin wrinkling. The salivary glands are affected as part of the generalized exocrine gland involvement. Clinically, the lips may be dry and swollen (Fig. **336**).

The differential diagnosis includes cheilitis glandularis, mucopolysaccharidosis, and lipoid proteinosis.

Laboratory test. Histopathologic examination of lip biopsy may confirm the diagnosis. Elevated levels of chloride and sodium in sweat and lack of pancreatic enzymes in the duodenal fluid are also helpful.

Treatment is supportive.

Histiocytosis X

Histiocytosis X is a histocytic proliferative disease that includes three entities of unknown cause: Letterer-Siwe disease, Hand-Schüller-Christian disease, and eosinophilic granuloma. Letterer-Siwe disease is the acute disseminated form, which usually appears during the first year of life and has a very poor prognosis. Clinically, it is characterized by fever, chills, hepatosplenomegaly, anemia, lymphadenopathy, osteolytic bone lesions, generalized skin rash (petechiae, scaly papules, nodules, vesicles, ulcers), and oral manifestations (Fig. **337**). The oral lesions are ulcers, ecchymoses, gingivitis, periodontitis, and loose teeth (Fig. **338**).

Hand-Schüller-Christian disease is the chronic disseminated form, which has a more benign course. It usually appears between 3 and 6 years of age and affects predominantly boys (2:1 ratio). Clinically, there is a classic triad consisting of osteolytic bone lesions (particularly of the skull), exophthalmos, and diabetes insipidus. This triad is present in only 25% of patients. Otitis media, a skin rash, and involvement of internal organs may also occur. The oral cavity is frequently involved in the early stages of the disease, with ulcers, edema, hyperplasia, and necrosis of the gingiva, halitosis, and bad taste (Fig. **339**). In cases of involvement of the jaw bones there is loosening of the teeth and severe periodontitis leading to loss of the teeth. Delayed healing of tooth sockets after extraction may be seen.

Eosinophilic granuloma is the localized benign form and usually affects adolescents or young adults. Males are affected more frequently than females. Clinically, the disease is characterized by asymptomatic monostotic or polyostotic osteolytic bone lesions, and on rare occasions there may be local edema and pain.

27. Precancerous Lesions

Leukoplakia

A precancerous lesion is defined by WHO as "a morphologically altered tissue in which cancer is more likely to occur than in its apparently normal counterpart." Oral leukoplakia is the most common and best studied precancerous lesion. Leukoplakia is a diagnosis by exclusion, and the term is now used in a clinical descriptive sense. It is defined as a white patch or plaque, firmly attached to the oral mucosa, that cannot be classified clinically and pathologically in any other disease entity. The available data show that the prevalence rate of leukoplakia ranges from 0.1 to 5% of the general population. The lesion seems to be more common in men than in women, especially between 40 and 60 years of age. The cause is still obscure. Some of the leukoplakias are tobacco-related, whereas in other cases predisposing factors, such as local irritation, Candida albicans, alcohol, industrial products, and possible viruses have been incriminated. However, it must be emphasized that nonsmokers with leukoplakia are at higher risk than smokers for development of cancer. Clinically, leukoplakia can be divided into two main forms: the homogeneous, which is common and characterized by an asymptomatic white homogeneous plaque with a smooth or wrinkled surface that occasionally may be traversed by fissures or cracks (Fig. 355), and the speckled or nodular form, which is rare and is characterized by a red base with multiple small white nodules or macules on which C. albicans infection is often superimposed (Fig. 356). In addition, two other clinical varieties of oral leukoplakia have been described: proliferative verrucous leukoplakia, which is rare and characterized by a white irregular exophytic papillary pattern (Fig. 357), is more common in females than males, shows a relatively prompt extension, and tends to reccur after surgical removal, and AIDS-related leukoplakia (hairy leukoplakia), which is a unique lesion in patients infected with human immunodeficiency virus (see p. 112). It is characterized initially by a slightly raised, poorly demarcated, and corrugated white patch with late formation of prominent projec-

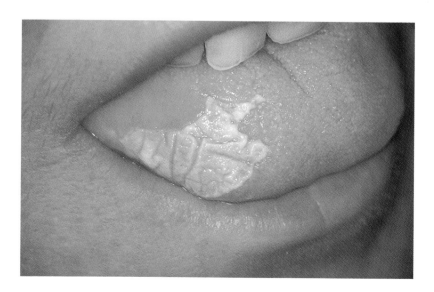

Fig. **355**. Homogeneous leukoplakia of the tongue.

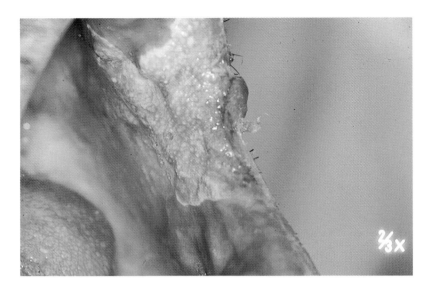

Fig. **356**. Speckled leukoplakia of the buccal mucosa.

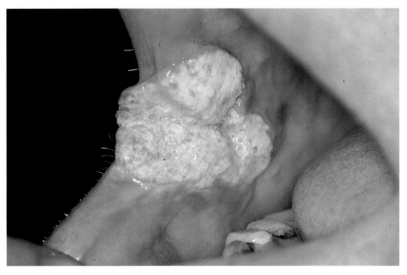

Fig. **357**. Proliferative verrucous leukoplakia of the buccal mucosa.

tions, and frequently it appears on the lateral borders of the tongue. This classification has practical clinical significance, since the speckled leukoplakia is four to five times more likely to result in malignant transformation than homogeneous leukoplakia. Proliferative verrucous leukoplakia also shows an increased risk, whereas the AIDS-related leukoplakia has not been described as progressing to malignancy.

Leukoplakia may occur at any site in the oral cavity. However, the most frequent locations are the buccal mucosa and commissures, followed by the tongue, palate, lip, alveolar mucosa, gingiva, and floor of the mouth (Figs. **358–365**). The lesions may be small or large and the sites of highest risk for development of a malignancy are the floor of the mouth, followed by the tongue and the lip. Clinical signs suggesting a potential malignancy are: speckled surface, erosion or ulceration in the lesion, development of a nodule, induration of the periphery, and the location of the lesion (high-risk sites). However, the aforementioned clinical criteria are not totally reliable and all lesions must be biopsied and subjected to rigorous microscopic examination. About 15 to 23% of clinical oral leukoplakia exhibits histologically epithelial dysplasia, carcinoma in situ, or invasive carcinoma at the time of initial biopsy. Follow-up studies of oral leukoplakia have found a frequency of malignant transformation ranging from 0.13 to 6%.

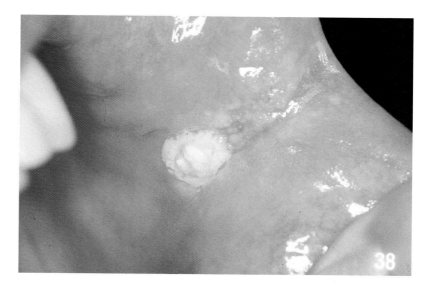

Fig. **358**. Leukoplakia of the buccal mucosa.

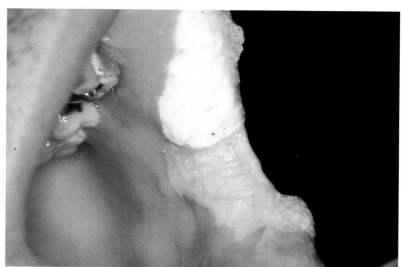

Fig. **359**. Leukoplakia of the buccal mucosa and commissure.

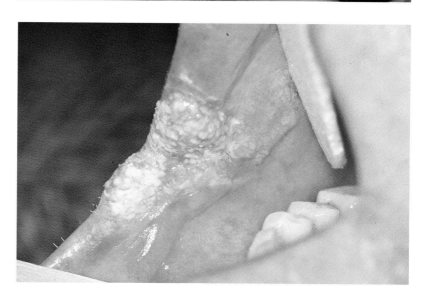

Fig. **360**. Speckled leukoplakia of the buccal mucosa and commissure.

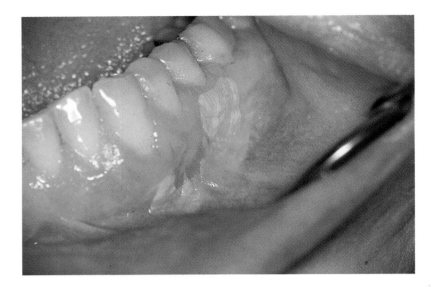

Fig. **361**. Leukoplakia of the alveolar mucosa.

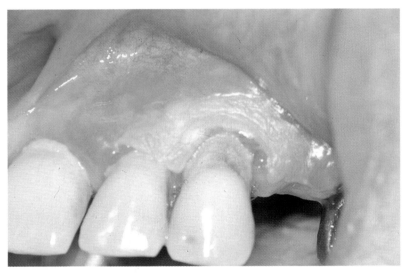

Fig. **362**. Leukoplakia of the gingiva.

The differential diagnosis includes hypertrophic lichen planus, chronic hyperplastic candidosis, chemical burn, leukoedema, discoid lupus erythematosus, and several genetic syndromes exhibiting disturbances of keratinization.

Laboratory test. Histopathologic examination is the most important test to define the nature and the relative risk of oral leukoplakic lesions. The presence of epithelial dysplasia signifies a precancerous lesion.

Treatment. Oral leukoplakia sometimes regresses after discontinuation of tobacco use. In addition, the elimination of any irritating factor is mandatory, and good oral hygiene and follow-up of the patients is indicated. Surgical excision is the treatment of choice. Recently, retinoic acid has been reported to be effective.

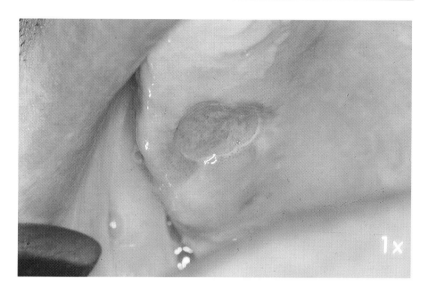

Fig. **416**. Acute myelocytic leukemia, ulcer on the palate.

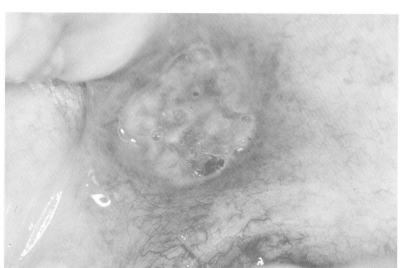

Fig. **417**. Acute lymphocytic leukemia, ulcer on the palate.

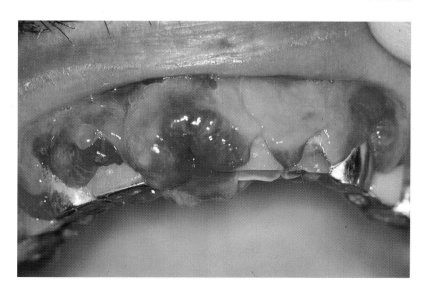

Fig. **418**. Acute myelomonocytic leukemia, severe gingival enlargement.

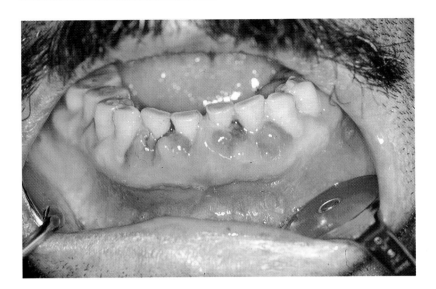

Fig. **419**. Acute myelocytic leukemia, marked gingival enlargement.

Chronic Leukemias

Chronic leukemias are classified into myelogenous and lymphocytic forms. They affect most frequently middle-aged persons. Men are more frequently affected than women.

The onset and course are usually insidious and the disease may be discovered accidentally during a routine blood check. Chronic malaise, fatigue, weight loss, night sweats, lymphadenopathy, splenomegaly and hepatomegaly, low-grade fever, enlargement of the parotid glands, and tenderness in the lower half of the sternum are common complaints. Skin manifestations include ecchymoses, petechiae, superficial ulcerations, papules, nodules, pruritus, and dark discoloration of the skin. Rarely, bullous pemphigoid or pemphigus may be associated with chronic leukemia.

The oral mucosa is less frequently affected than in acute leukemia. Clinically, there is pallor of the oral mucosa, petechiae, superficial ulceration, and bleeding episodes after routine oral surgery (Fig. **420**). Enlargement of the gingiva may occur in lymphocytic leukemia and less frequently in myelogenous leukemia (Figs. **421, 422**). Oral pemphigus and herpes zoster may also be associated with chronic leukemia.

The differential diagnosis includes trauma, agranulocytosis, thrombocytopenic purpura, aplastic anemia, cyclic neutropenia, gingivitis and periodontitis, idiopathic gingival fibromatosis, and gingival hyperplasia caused by phenytoin.

Laboratory tests helpful in establishing the diagnosis in all types of leukemia include peripheral blood count, bone marrow examination, and determination of various markers of the leukemic cells (histochemical, immunologic, etc.).

Treatment. A specialized team approach is required in the treatment of these disorders.

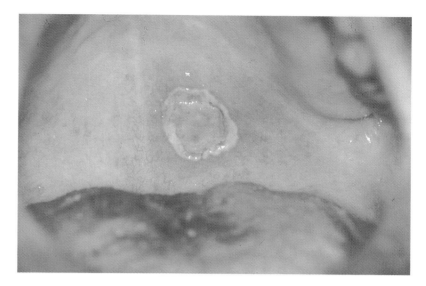

Fig. **420**. Chronic lymphocytic leukemia, ulcer on the palate.

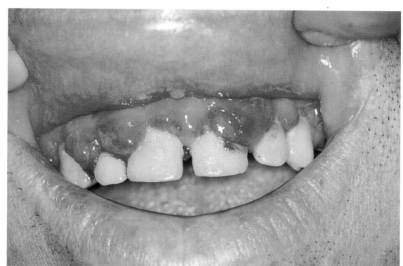

Fig. **421**. Chronic lymphocytic leukemia, severe gingival enlargement.

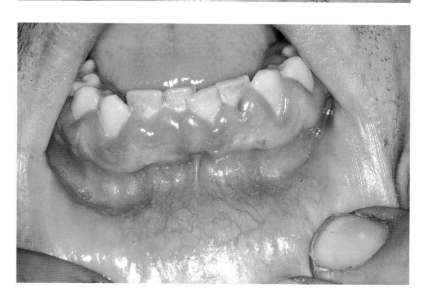

Fig. **422**. Chronic myelocytic leukemia, marked gingival enlargement.

Erythroleukemia

Erythroleukemia, or Di Guglielmo syndrome, is a variant of acute myelogenous leukemia. It represents about 3% of all cases of acute leukemia and is rare in childhood. During the early stages, it is characterized by intense erythroid proliferation in the bone marrow and abnormal red cells in the blood. This erythremic myelosis may evolve to either erythroleukemia or acute myelogenous leukemia. Clinically, there is anemia, fever, hepatosplenomegaly, and hemorrhages. The clinical course is downhill and resembles the course of acute myelomonocytic leukemia. The oral mucosa may rarely be affected, with gingival hemorrhages and enlargement (Fig. **423**).

Polycythemia Vera

Polycythemia vera is a relatively common myeloproliferative disorder characterized by an increase in the production of red cells and an absolute increase in erythroid mass. The cause remains obscure, and it is more common in men over 50 years of age. The disease usually has an insidious onset and is often discovered after a routine blood count that shows an elevated hemoglobin or hematocrit level. Clinically, it is characterized by headache, dizziness, vertigo, tinnitus, visual disturbances, cardiovascular and gastrointestinal symptoms, pruritus, hemorrhages, venous thromboses, and a ruddy cyanotic skin. The oral mucosa usually acquires a deep purplish red color (Fig. **424**). Gingival bleeding and enlargement, petechiae, and ecchymoses of the oral mucosa may also occur.

The differential diagnosis includes polycythemia secondary to various other causes, thrombocytopenic purpura, and other disorders of the blood platelets.

Laboratory tests helpful in establishing the diagnosis are the standard blood count and bone marrow examination.

Treatment is supportive and is best left to the specialist.

Hodgkin's Disease

Hodgkin's disease is a malignant disease of the mononuclear cell system rather than the lymphoid tissue per se. It is a disease of unknown cause that affects more often young males than females. Depending on the extent, Hodgkin's disease is classified as stage I, II, III, or IV and further characterized as A or B, depending on absence or presence of systemic manifestations. This staging along with the histologic typing of the disease determines the treatment and the prognosis. Painless enlargement of cervical lymph nodes or other groups of lymph nodes is a common manifestation (Fig. **425**). Anorexia, weight loss, fever, night sweats, and pruritus may accompany lymphadenopathy early in the course of the disease, or alternatively these systemic manifestations may appear later. If the disease metastasizes to extra lymphatic tissues, a constellation of symptoms and signs appears, depending on the site of metastasis and the organ involved.

A variety of skin manifestations may be associated with Hodgkin's disease, such as erythema nodosum, exfoliative dermatitis, pemphigus, dermatomyositis.

The oral cavity is an infrequent site of metastatic Hodgkin's disease, where ulcers or red swollen areas may appear (Fig. **426**). However, submandibular and cervical lymphadenopathy are common initial signs. The involved nodes are multiple or solitary, bilateral or unilateral, and rubbery on palpation.

The differential diagnosis includes non-Hodgkin's lymphomas, necrotizing sialometaplasia, squamous cell carcinoma, Wegener's granulomatosis, lethal midline granuloma, and infectious mononucleosis.

Laboratory tests helpful in establishing the diagnosis are histopathologic examination of involved lymph nodes or biopsy of lesions that appear suspicious.

Treatment. Radiotherapy and chemotherapy.

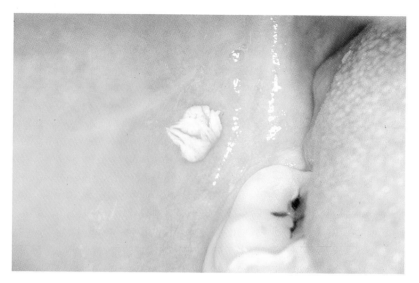

Fig. **435**. Papilloma of the buccal mucosa.

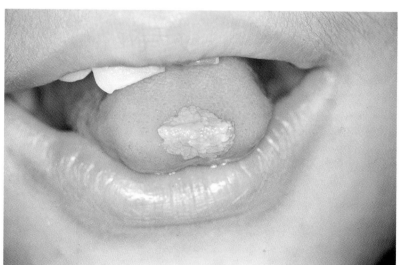

Fig. **436**. Papilloma of the tongue.

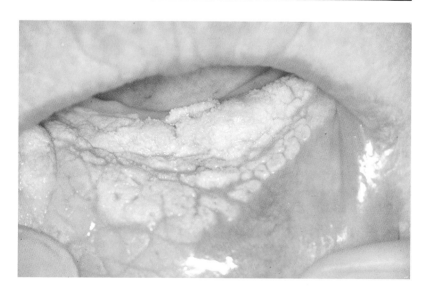

Fig. **437**. Verrucous hyperplasia of the alveolar and lip mucosa.

Keratoacanthoma

Keratoacanthoma is a fairly common benign skin tumor that probably arises from the hair follicles. The tumor occurs on exposed skin, especially the face. It is more common in men than women (ratio 1.8:1) and is usually seen in persons more than 50 years of age. Clinically, it appears as a painless well-circumscribed dome or bud-shaped tumor of 1 to 2 cm diameter, with a keratin crater at the center. The tumor begins as a small nodule that grows rapidly and, within 4 to 8 weeks, reaches its full size. For a period of 1 to 2 months, it persists without change, and then it may undergo spontaneous regression over the next 5 to 10 weeks. About 10% of keratoacanthomas are located on the lips (Fig. **438**), whereas very few cases have been reported intraorally (Fig. **439**).

Based on the histogenesis and the biologic behavior, two types of keratoacanthoma are now recognized. Type I (bud-shaped) arises as a result of thickening and elongation of the walls of the superficial parts of hair follicles. Type II (dome-shaped) arises from the deeper part of the hair follicles or hair germ.

The differential diagnosis should include basal and squamous cell carcinomas and warty dyskeratoma.

Laboratory test. The diagnosis is based on histopathologic examination.

Treatment. Although some keratoacanthomas regress spontaneously, for esthetic reasons the treatment of choice is surgical excision, or radiation in small doses.

Fibroma

Fibroma is the most common benign tumor of the oral cavity and originates from the connective tissue. It is believed that the true fibroma is very rare and that most cases represent fibrous hyperplasia caused by chronic irritation. It occurs in both sexes, most often between the ages of 30 and 50 years. Clinically, the fibroma is a well-defined, firm, sessile or pedunculated tumor with a smooth surface of normal epithelium (Fig. **440**). It appears as an asymptomatic, single lesion usually under 1 cm in diameter, although in rare cases it may reach several centimeters. It often occurs on the gingiva, buccal mucosa, lips, tongue, and palate.

The differential diagnosis includes giant cell fibroma, lipoma, myxoma, peripheral ossifying fibroma, neurofibroma, schwannoma, fibrous histiocytoma, fibrous hyperplasia of the tuberosity, and pleomorphic adenoma.

Laboratory test. Histopathologic examination is essential for the diagnosis.

Treatment is surgical excision.

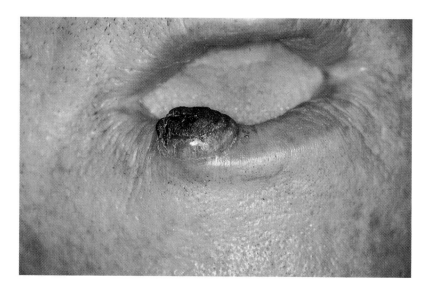

Fig. **438**. Keratoacanthoma of the vermilion border of the lower lip.

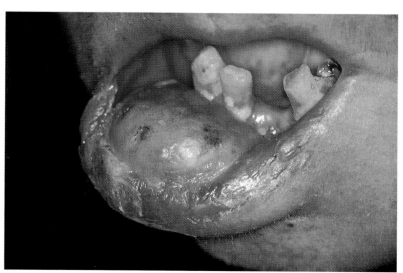

Fig. **439**. Keratoacanthoma of the lower lip mucosa.

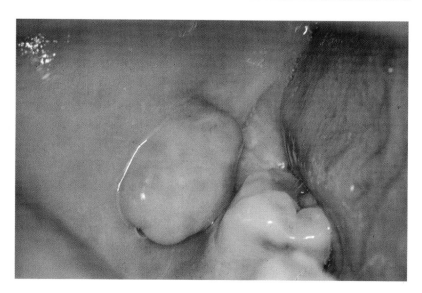

Fig. **440**. Fibroma of the buccal mucosa.

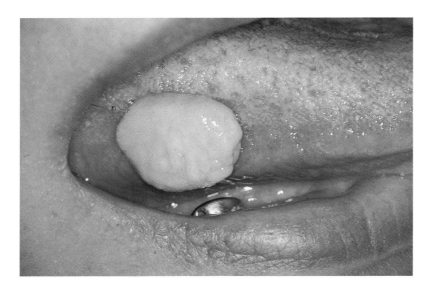

Fig. **441**. Giant cell fibroma of the tongue.

Giant Cell Fibroma

Giant cell fibroma is a fibrous lesion of the oral mucosa that is histologically characterized by the presence of numerous stellate and multinucleated cells. Clinically, it presents as a painless well-circumscribed and pedunculated tumor with a normal color and slightly nodular surface (Fig. **441**). The lesion varies in size from a few millimeters to 1 cm.

The giant cell fibroma is more common during the first three decades of life and displays a marked predilection for the gingiva, followed by the tongue, palate, buccal mucosa, and lip.

The differential diagnosis should include fibroma, neurofibroma, papilloma, peripheral ossifying fibroma, and pyogenic granuloma.

Laboratory test. The diagnosis is made on histopathologic criteria.

Treatment is surgical excision.

Peripheral Ossifying Fibroma

Peripheral ossifying fibroma, or peripheral odontogenic fibroma, is a benign tumor that is located exclusively on the gingiva and has characteristic histomorphologic features. The exact origin is unknown, although it is believed that it derives from the periodontal ligament. It is more common in children and young adults and has a predilection for females (ratio 1.7:1). Clinically, it is a well-defined firm tumor, sessile or pedunculated, covered by smooth normal epithelium (Figs. **442**, **443**). Usually the surface is ulcerated due to me-

chanical trauma. The size varies from a few millimeters to 1 to 2 cm, and more than 50% of the lesions occur in the incisor-cuspid region in both jaws.

The differential diagnosis should include traumatic fibroma, giant cell fibroma, peripheral giant cell granuloma, pyogenic granuloma, and pregnancy granuloma.

Laboratory test. The diagnosis is based on histopathologic criteria.

Treatment is surgical excision.

Lipoma

Lipoma is a benign tumor of adipose tissue relatively rare in the oral cavity. It is more common between 40 and 60 years of age and is usually located on the buccal mucosa, tongue, mucobuccal fold, floor of the mouth, lips, and gingiva. Clinically, it appears as a painless, well-defined tumor, pedunculated or sessile, varying in size from a few millimeters to several centimeters of yellowish or pink color (Fig. **444**). The covering epithelium is thin, with visible blood vessels. It is soft on palpation and occasionally fluctuant and may be misdiagnosed as a cyst, especially when it is located in the deeper submucosal tissues.

The differential diagnosis includes myxoma, fibroma, mucocele, and small dermoid cyst.

Laboratory test. The diagnosis is established by histopathologic examination.

Treatment is surgical excision.

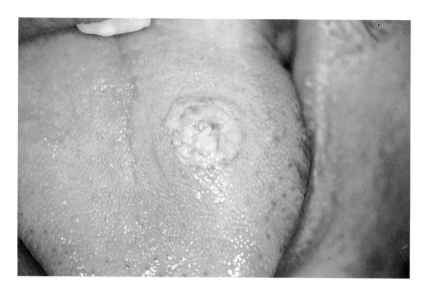

Fig. **452**. Benign fibrous histiocytoma on the dorsum of the tongue.

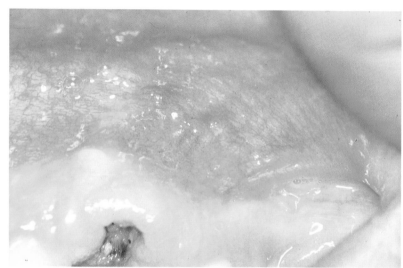

Fig. **453**. Capillary hemangioma.

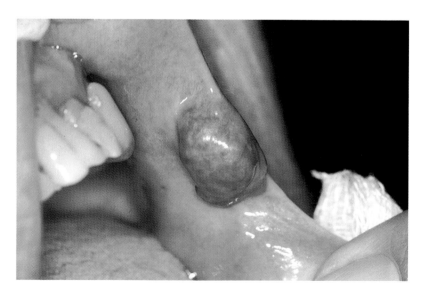

Fig. **454**. Cavernous hemangioma.

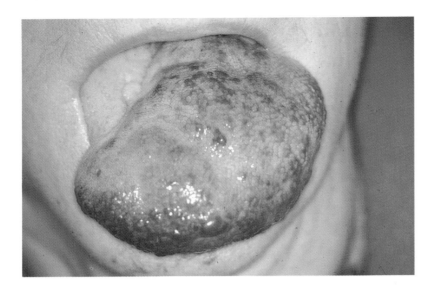

Fig. **455**. Extensive hemangioma of the tongue.

common sites on involvement. The size ranges from a few millimeters to extensive lesions (Fig. 455), which may cause organ deformities (such as macroglossia, macrocheilia). Rarely, hemangiomas may develop in the jaw bones.

The differential diagnosis includes pyogenic granuloma, hemangioendothelioma, hemangiopericytoma, Kaposi's sarcoma and several syndromes with oral vascular lesions, such as the Sturge-Weber syndrome, Maffucci's syndrome, Klippel-Trenaunay-Weber syndrome, and the Rendu-Osler-Weber syndrome.

Laboratory test useful for the diagnosis is histopathologic examination. The biopsy has to be taken very cautiously because of the danger of hemorrhage.

The treatment is surgical excision or cryotherapy or injection of sclerosing agents into the lesion. Some congenital hemangiomas have been found to undergo spontaneous regression.

Lymphangioma

Lymphangioma is a relatively common benign tumor of the oral cavity and, like hemangioma, it is a developmental abnormality rather than a true neoplasm. The great majority of the lesions appear during the first 3 years of life and show a marked predilection for the head and neck region. Clinically, oral lymphangiomas are characterized by small soft elevated nodules that resemble small cysts and have normal, or yellow-grayish or red

color (Figs. **456, 457**). If the lesion is located deeper in the oral tissues, it appears as a diffuse mass without change of color. The size ranges from a few millimeters to extremely large lesions that cause organ deformities (Fig. **458**). The dorsum of the tongue is the most frequent site of involvement. Less often, it may be found on the lips, buccal mucosa, floor of the mouth and soft palate, but it is extremely rare on the gingiva. It is usually asymptomatic, but when it gets larger, it may cause pain and discomfort during speech, chewing, and swallowing, or macroglossia. Recurrent infection of the lesion is common and constitutes a serious problem.

The differential diagnosis includes hemangioma, median rhomboid glossitis, lingual thyroid, and papillary hyperplasia of the palate. Deep lymphangiomas may be confused with other mesenchymal neoplasms.

Laboratory test. Histopathologic examination is essential for diagnosis.

Treatment is surgical excision.

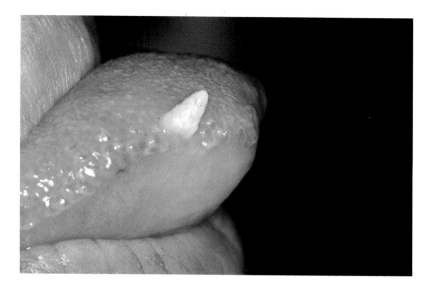

Fig. **463**. Mucosal horn on the tongue.

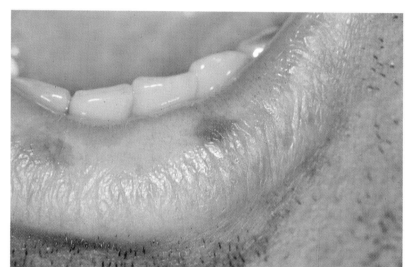

Fig. **464**. Freckles on the vermilion border of the lower lip.

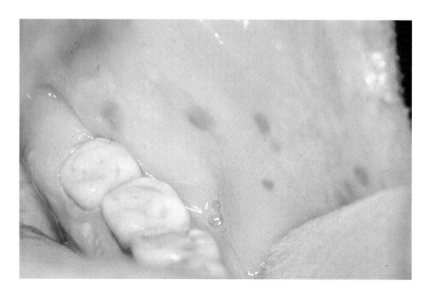

Fig. **465**. Lentigo of the buccal mucosa.

Intramucosal Nevus

Pigmented cellular nevi are developmental malformations originating from defective melanoblasts of the neural crest. They usually occur in the skin and rarely in the oral mucosa. They are collections of nevus cells in the epidermis, dermis, or both. There are two main varieties of nevi: congenital and acquired. Based on histologic criteria (location of nevus cells and the presence or absence of junctional activity), acquired nevi may be divided into many categories. In the oral mucosa four types have been described: the intramucosal, junctional, compound, and blue. The intramucosal nevus is more common, representing 55% of the oral nevi. It consists of a number of nevus cells that are embedded in the connective tissue and are separated from the epithelium by a band of collagen. It is more common in females and may be found at any age. Clinically, it is an asymptomatic, flat, or slightly elevated spot or plaque of brown or brown-black color (Fig. **466**). It is usually located on the palate and buccal mucosa and rarely on the gingiva and the lips. Intramucosal nevi have little capacity for malignant transformation.

The differential diagnosis includes other types of oral nevi, freckles, lentigo simplex, amalgam tattoo, hematoma, lentigo maligna, and malignant melanoma.

Laboratory test. The diagnosis is established by histopathologic examination.

Treatment. Usually no treatment is required. However, surgical excision is recommended when the nevus is located at a site of chronic irritation or exhibits any change in its appearance.

Junctional Nevus

Junctional nevus is the least frequent of oral nevi, accounting for about 3 to 5.5% of the cases. Histologically, it is characterized by nests of nevus cells along the basal layer of the epithelium. Some of these cells drop off into the underlying connective tissue, showing junctional activity. The clinical features of junctional nevus are not pathognomonic. They appear typically as asymptomatic black or brown flat or slightly elevated spots, which have a diameter of 0.1 to 0.5 cm (Fig. **467**). It is found more often on the palate, buccal mucosa, and alveolar mucosa. The junctional nevus has a significant capacity to undergo malignant transformation into melanoma. Clinically,

any change in color, size, and texture of an oral nevus should be regarded with suspicion and the possibility of malignant melanoma should not be excluded.

The differential diagnosis includes the other types of oral nevi, freckles, lentigo simplex, amalgam tattoo, normal pigmentation, lentigo maligna, and malignant melanoma.

Laboratory test. The diagnosis is made exclusively on histologic criteria.

Treatment is surgical excision.

Compound Nevus

Compound nevus is characterized by clusters of nevus cells located both in the epithelium and in the underlying connective tissue; therefore it has the characteristics of both intramucosal and junctional nevus. Compound nevus is rare in the oral cavity, representing about 6 to 8.5% of all oral nevi. There is no sex or age predilection. Clinically, it appears as an asymptomatic slightly elevated or flat spot that has red-brown or black-brown color, and the size varies from a few millimeters to 1 cm in diameter (Fig. **468**). It is more often located on the buccal mucosa, the palate, and the gingiva. Compound nevi may be transformed into malignant melanoma.

The differential diagnosis should include other oral nevi, lentigo simplex, freckles, lentigo maligna, amalgam tattoo, and malignant melanoma.

Laboratory test. The diagnosis is exclusively made by histologic examination.

Treatment is the same as for intramucosal nevus.

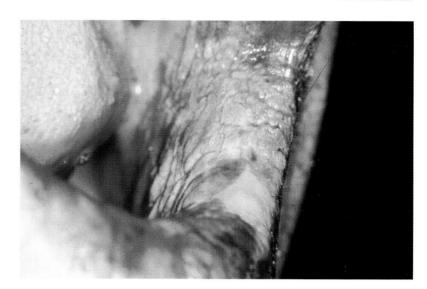

Fig. **472**. Lentigo maligna on the buccal mucosa, commissure, and lower lip.

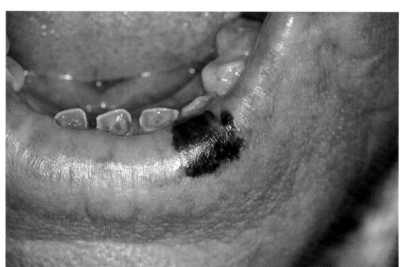

Fig. **473**. Lentigo maligna on the vermilion border of the lower lip.

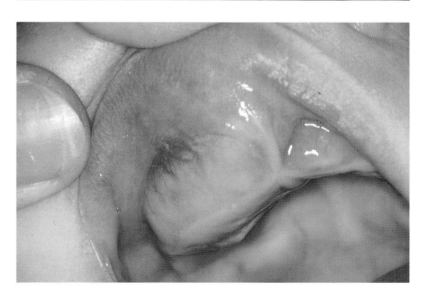

Fig. **474**. Melanotic neuroectodermal tumor of infancy in the maxilla.

Pleomorphic Adenoma

Pleomorphic adenoma is the most common benign neoplasm of the major and minor salivary glands. It represents 62.6 to 75.6% of all tumors of major salivary glands and 42.6 to 70% of all minor salivary gland tumors. The posterior part of the palate is the usual intraoral site of involvement, followed by the upper lip, retromolar area, buccal mucosa, and tongue (Figs. **475, 476**). About 90% of the cases of major salivary gland tumors occur in the parotid gland. Pleomorphic adenoma has no significant sex predilection and occurs more often between 40 and 70 years of age. When located in the minor salivary glands, it is an asymptomatic slow-growing firm swelling, with a size of 2 to 3 cm in diameter. The tumor is covered by normal epithelium and is rarely ulcerated. It may cause difficulties in chewing, speech, and fitting a denture.

The differential diagnosis includes other salivary gland tumors, lipoma, and necrotizing sialometaplasia.

Laboratory test. The diagnosis is made by histologic examination.

Treatment is surgical excision.

Papillary Cystadenoma Lymphomatosum

Papillary cystadenoma lymphomatosum, or adenolymphoma or Warthin's tumor, is a rare benign tumor of the salivary glands, almost always located in the parotid gland. However, it is occasionally observed in the submandibular gland and the intraoral minor salivary glands. The tumor is more frequent in men than women of 40 to 70 years of age, and the most common intraoral location is the palate and the lips. Clinically, it is a painless slow-growing firm superficial swelling, with size that varies from 1 to 4 cm in diameter (Fig. **477**).

The differential diagnosis includes other benign and malignant salivary gland tumors, branchial cyst, and tuberculous lymphadenopathy.

Laboratory test. The diagnosis is made by histologic examination.

Treatment is surgical excision.

Budtz-Jørgensen E: The significance of Candida albicans in denture stomatitis. Scand J Dent Res 82:151, 1974.

Cawson BA, Lehner T: Chronic hyperplastic candidiasis – Candida leukoplakia. Br J Dermatol 80:9, 1968.

Epstein JB, Pearsall NN, Truelove EL: Oral candidiasis: Effect of antifungal therapy upon clinical sign and symptoms, salivary antibody and mucosal adherence of Candida albicans. Oral Surg 51:32, 1981.

Eyre J, Nally FF: Oral cándidosis and carcinoma. Br J Dermatol 85:73, 1971.

Farman AG, Nutt G: Oral Candida, debilitating disease and atrophic lesions of the tongue. J Biol Buccale 4:203, 1976.

Higgs JM, Wells RS: Chronic mucocutaneous candidiasis: Associated abnormalities of iron metabolism. Br J Dermatol 86 (Suppl 8):88, 1972.

Holbrook WP, Rodgers GD: Candidal infections: Experience in a British dental hospital. Oral Surg 49:122, 1980.

Holmstrup P, Bessermann M: Clinical, therapeutic and pathogenic aspects of chronic oral multifocal candidiasis. Oral Surg 56:388, 1983.

Kirkpatrick CH, Sohnle PG: Chronic mucocutaneous candidiasis. In: Safai B, Good RA, (eds): Immunodermatology. Plenum Press, New York, 1981, p 495.

Klein RS, Harris CA, Small CB, et al: Oral candidiasis in high-risk patients as the initial manifestation of the acquired immunodeficiency syndrome. N Engl J Med 311:354, 1984.

Kolnick JR: Oral candidosis. Oral Surg 50:411, 1980.

Lehner T: Oral candidosis. Dent Pract 17:209, 1967.

Mac Farlane TW, Helnarska SJ: The microbiology of angular cheilitis. Br Dent J 140:403, 1976.

Miller RL, Gould AR, Skolnick JL, Epstein WM: Localized oral histoplasmosis. Oral Surg 53:367, 1982.

Mylbarniemi S, Perheentura J: Oral findings in the autoimmune polyendocrinopathy-candidosis syndrome and other forms of hypoparathyroidism. Oral Surg 45:721, 1978.

Page LR, Drummond JF, Daniels HT, et al: Blastomycosis with oral lesions. Oral Surg 47:157, 1979.

Renner RP, Lee M, Andors L, Mc Namara TF: The role of Candida albicans in denture stomatitis. Oral Surg 47:323, 1979.

Rockoff AS: Chronic mucocutaneous candidiasis. Arch Dermatol 115:322, 1979.

Samaranayake LP, Mc Farlane TW: A retrospective study of patients with recurrent chronic atrophic candidosis. Oral Surg 52:150, 1981.

Silverman S Jr, Migliorati CA, Lozanda-Nur F, et al: Oral findings in people with or at high risk for AIDS: A study of 375 homosexual males. J Am Dent Assoc 112:187, 1986.

Tavitian A, Raufman J-P, Rosenthal LE: Oral candidiasis as a marker for esophageal candidiasis in the acquired immunodeficiency syndrome. Ann Intern Med 104:54, 1986.

Toth BB, Frame RR: Oral histoplasmosis: Diagnostic complication and treatment. Oral Surg 55:597, 1983.

Witorsch P, Utz JP: North American blastomycosis: A study of 40 patients. Medicine (Baltimore) 47:169, 1968.

Wright BA, Fenwick F: Candidiasis and atrophic tongue lesions. Oral Surg 51:55, 1981.

Yusuf H, Craig GT, Allan D: Disseminated histoplasmosis presenting with oral lesions. Br J Oral Surg 16:234, 1978–79.

18. Other Infections

DeLuke DM, Sciubba JJ: Oral manifestations of sarcoidosis: Report of a case masquerading as a neoplasm. Oral Surg 59:184, 1985.

Farah FS, Malac JA: Cutaneous leishmaniasis. Arch Dermatol 103:467, 1971.

Farah FS: Protozoan and helminth infections, in: Fitzpatrick TB, Eisen AZ, Wolff K, et al, (eds): Dermatology in General Medicine, 3rd ed. Mc Graw-Hill, New York, 1987, p 2480.

Gold RS, Flanders NJ, Sager E: Oral sarcoidosis: Review of the literature. J Oral Surg 34:237, 1976.

Greer RO, Sanger RG: Primary intraoral sarcoidosis. J Oral Surg 35:507, 1977.

Hamner JE, Scofield HH: Cervical lymphadenopathy and parotid gland swelling in sarcoidosis. J Am Dent Assoc 74:1224, 1967.

James DG, Jones WW: Immunology of sarcoidosis. Am J Med 72:5, 1982.

Orlian AI, Birnbaum M: Intraoral localized sarcoid lesion. Oral Surg 49:341, 1980.

Sloan PJM, O'Neil TCA, Smith CJ, Holdsworth CD: Multisystem sarcoid presenting with gingival hyperplasia. Br J Oral Surg 21:31, 1983.

Verheijen-Breemhaar L, DeMan K, Zondervan PE, Hilvering C: Sarcoidosis with maxillary involvement. Int J Oral Maxillofac Surg 16:104, 1987.

19. Diseases with Possible Immunopathogenesis

Basu MK, Asquith P, Thompson RA, Cooke WT: Oral manifestations of Crohn's disease. Gut 16:249, 1975.

Bernstein ML, McDonald JS: Oral lesions in Crohn's disease: Report of two cases and update of the literature. Oral Surg 46:234, 1978.

Brook IM, King DJ, Miller ID: Chronic granulomatous cheilitis and its relationship to Crohn's disease. Oral Surg 56:405, 1983.

Brooke RI, Sapp JP: Herpetiform ulceration. Oral Surg 42:182, 1976.

Butler DJ, Thompson H: Malignant granuloma. Br J Oral Surg 9:208, 1972.

Catterall RD: Clinical aspects of Reiter's disease. Br J Rheumat 22:151, 1983.

Challacombe SJ, Barkhan P, Lehner T: Haematological features and differentiation of recurrent oral ulceration. Br J Oral Surg 15:37, 1977–78.

Cohen PS, Meltzer JA: Strawberry gums: A sign of Wegener's granulomatosis. JAMA 246:2610, 1981.

Crama-Bohbouth G, Bosman FT, Vermeer BJ, et al: Immunohistological findings in lip biopsy specimens from patients with Crohn's disease and healthy subjects. Gut 24:202, 1983.

Edwards MB, Buckerfield JP: Wegener's granulomatosis: A case with primary mucocutaneous lesions. Oral Surg 46:53, 1978.

Frankel DH, Mostofi RS, Lorincz AL: Oral Crohn's disease: Report of two cases in brothers with metallic dysgeusia and a review of the literature. J Am Acad Dermatol 12:260, 1985.

Freiberger HF, Fudenberg HH: Behçet's disease: Pitfalls in therapy and diagnosis. Hosp Pract 15:49g, 1980.

Gallina G, Cumbo V, Messina P, Caruso C: HLA-A,B,C,DR,MT and MB antigens in recurrent aphthous stomatitis. Oral Surg 59:364, 1985.

Greenspan JS, Gadol N, Olson JA, et al: Lymphocyte function in recurrent aphthous ulceration. J Oral Pathol 14:592, 1985.

Haim S, Gilhar A: Clinical and laboratory criteria for the diagnosis of Behçet's disease. Br J Dermatol 102:361, 1980.

Ishii Y, Yamanaka N, Ogawa K, et al: Nasal T-cell lymphoma as a type of so-called "lethal midline granuloma." Cancer 50:2336, 1982.

Keczkes K: Wegener's granulomatosis. Combined therapy with low-dose systemic corticosteroids, azathioprine and cyclophosphamide in three patients. Br J Dermatol 94:391, 1976.

Kousa M: Clinical observations on Reiter's disease with special reference to the venereal and non-venereal aetiology. Acta Derm Venereol [Suppl] (Stockh) 58:18, 1978.

Lehner T: Fine structural findings in recurrent oral ulceration. Br Dent J 121:454, 1966.

Lehner T: Pathology of recurrent oral ulceration and oral ulceration in Behçet syndrome: Light, electron and fluorescence microscopy. J Pathol 97:481, 1969.

Lehner T: Immunologic aspects of recurrent oral ulcers. Oral Surg 33:80, 1972.

Lehner T: Progress report. Oral ulceration and Behçet's syndrome. Gut 18:491, 1977.

Lennette HE, Magoffin R: Virologic and immunologic aspects of major oral ulceration. J Am Dent Assoc 87:1055, 1973.

Miller MF, Garfunkel AA, Ram CA, Ship II: The inheritance of recurrent aphthous stomatitis. Oral Surg 49:409, 1980.

Nelson JF, Finkelstein MW, Acevedo A, et al: Midline "nonhealing" granuloma. Oral Surg 58:554, 1984.

Pindborg JJ, Gorlin RJ, Asboe-Hansen G: Reiter's syndrome. Review of the literature and report of a case. Oral Surg 16:551, 1963.

Savage NW, Seymour GJ, Kruger BJ: Expression of class I and class II major histocompatibility complex antigens on epithelial cells in recurrent aphthous stomatitis. J Oral Pathol 15:191, 1986.

Sharp JT: Reiter's syndrome: A review of current status and a hypothesis regarding its pathogenesis. Curr Probl Dermatol 5:157, 1973.

Sun A, Wu Y-C, Liang L-C, Kwan H-W: Circulating immune complexes in recurrent oral ulcers. J Dermatol 13:170, 1986.

Taylor VE, Smith CJ: Oral manifestations of Crohn's disease without demonstrable gastrointestinal lesions. Oral Surg 39:58, 1975.

Tsokos M, Fauci AS, Costa J: Idiopathic midline destructive disease (IMDD): A subgroup of patients with the "midline granuloma" syndrome. Am J Clin Pathol 77:162, 1982.

Tyldesley WR: Oral Crohn's disease and related conditions. Br J Oral Surg 17:1, 1979–80.

20. Autoimmune (Collagen) Diseases

Berdon JK, Girasole RV: Oral manifestations of lupoid hepatitis. Oral Surg 33:900, 1972.

Callen JP: The value of malignancy evaluation in patients with dermatomyositis. J Am Acad Dermatol 6:253, 1982.

Green D: Scleroderma and its oral manifestations. Report of three cases of progressive systemic sclerosis (diffuse scleroderma). Oral Surg 15:1312, 1962.

Hidano A, Kaneko K, Arai Y, Kikuchi R: Survey of the prognosis for dermatomyositis, with special refference to its association with malignancy and pulmonary fibrosis. J Dermatol 13:233, 1986.

Jonsson R, Heyden G, Westberg NG, Nyberg G: Oral mucosal lesions in systemic lupus erythematosus. A clinical, histopathological and immunopathological study. J Rheumatol 11:38, 1984.

Marmary Y, Glaiss A, Pisanty S: Scleroderma: Oral manifestations. Oral Surg 52:32, 1981.

Moutsopoulos HM, Webber BL, Vlagopoulos TP, et al: Differences in the clinical manifestations of sicca syndrome in the presence and absence of rheumatoid arthritis. Am J Med 66:733, 1979.

Moutsopoulos HM, et al: Sjögren's syndrome (sicca syndrome): Current issues. Ann Intern Med 92:212, 1980.

Naylor WP: Oral management of the scleroderma patients. J Am Dent Assoc 105:814, 1982.

Rowell N, Hopper F: The periodontal membrane in systemic sclerosis. Br J Dermatol 96:15, 1977.

Sanger RG, Kirby JW: The oral and facial manifestations of dermatomyositis with calcinosis. Oral Surg 35:476, 1973.

Schiødt M: Oral manifestations of lupus erythematosus. Int J Oral Surg 13:101, 1984.

Schiødt M, Pindborg JJ: Oral discoid lupus erythematosus. I. The validity of previous histopathologic diagnostic criteria. Oral Surg 57:46, 1984.

Scully C: Sjögren's syndrome: Clinical and laboratory features, immunophogenesis and management. Oral Surg 62:510, 1986.

Sherlock S: Diseases of the Liver and Biliary System, 5th ed. Blackwell Scientific Publications, Oxford, 1975.

Weisman RA, Calcaterra TC: Head and neck manifestations of scleroderma. Ann Otol 87:332, 1978.

Wright JM, Dunsworth AR: Follicular lymphoid hyperplasia of the hard palate: A benign lymphoproliferative process. Oral Surg 55:162, 1983.

21. Skin Diseases

Aboobaker J, Bhogal B, Wojnarowska F, et al: The localization of the binding site of circulating IgA antibodies in linear IgA disease of adults, chronic bullous disease of childhood and childhood cicatricial pemphigoid. Br J Dermatol 116:293, 1987.

Barnett ML, Wittwer JW, Miller RL: Desquamative gingivitis in a 13-year-old male: Case report. J Periodontol 52:270, 1981.

Brown J, Winkelmann RK: Acanthosis nigricans: A study of 90 cases. Medicine (Baltimore) 47:33, 1968.

Buchner A, Begleiter A: Oral lesions in psoriatic patients. Oral Surg 41:327, 1976.

Buchner A, Lozada F, Silverman S: Histopathologic spectrum of oral erythema multiforme. Oral Surg 49:221, 1980.

Buckley DB, English J, Molloy W, et al: Dermatitis herpetiformis: A review of 119 cases. Clin Exp Dermatol 8:477, 1983.

Bystryn JC: Adjuvant therapy of pemphigus. Arch Dermatol 120:941, 1984.

Cataldo E, Mc Carthy P, Yaffee H: Psoriasis with oral manifestations. Cutis 20:705, 1977.

Caughman SW: Epidermolysis bullosa acquisita. Arch Dermatol 122:159, 1986.

Chau MNY, Radden BG: Oral warty dyskeratoma. J Oral Pathol 13:546, 1984.

Cohen HJ: Perioral dermatitis. J Am Acad Dermatol 4:739, 1981.

Curth HO: The necessity of distinguishing four types of acanthosis nigricans. Proceedings of the XIII International Congress of Dermatology, vol I, p 557, 1968.

Dean AG, Melish ME, Hicks R, Palumbo NE: An epidemic of Kawasaki syndrome in Hawaii. J Pediatr 100:552, 1982.

Economopoulou P, Laskaris G: Dermatitis herpetiformis: Oral lesions as an early manifestation. Oral Surg 62:77, 1986.

Epstein O: Lichen planus and liver disease. Br J Dermatol 111:473, 1984.

Farber EM, Nall ML: The natural history of psoriasis in 5,600 patients. Dermatologica 148:1, 1974.

Fraser NG, Kerr NW, Donald D: Oral lesions in dermatitis herpetiformis. Br J Dermatol 89:439, 1973.

Furue M, Iwata M, Tamaki K, Ishibashi Y: Anatomical distribution and immunological characteristics of epidermolysis bullosa acquisita antigen and bullous pemphigoid antigen. Br J Dermatol 114:651, 1986.

Gallgher G, Shklar G: Oral involvement in mucous membrane pemphigoid. Clin Dermatol 5:18, 1987.

Giallorenzi A, Goldstein B: Acute (toxic) epidermal necrolysis. Oral Surg 40:611, 1975.

Imamura S, Yanase K, Taniguchi S, et al: Erythema multiforme: Demonstration of immune complexes in the sera and skin lesions. Br J Dermatol 102:161, 1980.

Jablonska S, Chorzelski TP, Blaszczyk M, Maciejowska E: Bullous diseases and malignancy. Semin Dermatol 3:316, 1984.

Jordon RE, Kawana S, Fritz KA: Immunopathologic mechanisms in pemphigus and bullous pemphigoid. J Invest Dermatol 85:72s, 1985.

Kanerva L, Hietanen J: Ultrastructure of oral mucous membrane lesions in psoriasis. Acta Derm Venereol (Stockh) 64:191, 1984.

Kato S, Kimura M, Tsuji K, et al: HLA antigens in Kawasaki disease. Pediatrics 61:252, 1978.

Katz SI, Strober W: The pathogenesis of dermatitis herpetiformis. J Invest Dermatol 70:63, 1978.

Kawasaki T, Kosaki F, Okawa S, et al: A new infantile acute febrile mucocutaneous lymph node syndrome (MLNS) prevailing in Japan. Pediatrics 54:271, 1974.

Kazmierowski J, Wuepper K: Erythema multiforme: Immune complex vasculitis of the superficial cutaneous microvasculature. J Invest Dermatol 71:366, 1978.

Langeland T: Childhood cicatricial pemphigoid with linear IgA deposits: A case report. Acta Derm Venereol (Stockh) 65:354, 1985.

Laskaris G, Papavasiliou S, Bovopoulou O, Nicolis G: Association of oral pemphigus with chronic lymphocytic leukemia. Oral Surg 50:244, 1980.

Laskaris G: Oral pemphigus vulgaris: An immunofluorescent study of 58 cases. Oral Surg 51:626, 1981.

Laskaris G, Sklavounou A, Bovopoulou O: Juvenile pemphigus vulgaris. Oral Surg 51:415, 1981.

Laskaris G, Angelopoulos A: Cicatricial pemphigoid: Direct and indirect immunofluorescent studies. Oral Surg 51:48, 1981.

Laskaris G, Papavasiliou S, Bovopoulou O, Nicolis G: Lichen planus pigmentosus of the oral mucosa: A rare clinical variety. Dermatologica 162:61, 1981.

Laskaris G, Papanicolaou S, Angelopoulos A: Immunofluorescent study of cytologic smears in oral pemphigus: A simple diagnostic technique. Oral Surg 51:531, 1981.

Laskaris G, Sklavounou A, Angelopoulos A: Direct immunofluorescence in oral lichen planus. Oral Surg 53:483, 1982.

Laskaris G, Sklavounou A, Stratigos J: Bullous pemphigoid, cicatricial pemphigoid and pemphigus vulgaris. A comparative clinical study of 278 cases. Oral Surg 54:656, 1982.

Laskaris G, Sklavounou A: Warty dyskeratoma of the oral mucosa. Br J Oral Maxillofac Surg 23:371, 1985.

Laskaris G, Triantafyllou A, Economopoulou P: Gingival manifestations of childhood cicatricial pemphigoid. Oral Surg 1988. In press.

Leonard JN, Haffenden GP, Ring NP, et al: Linear IgA disease in adults. Br J Dermatol 107:301, 1982.

Leonard JN, Wright P, Williams DM, et al: The relationship between linear IgA disease and benign mucous membrane pemphigoid. Br J Dermatol 110:307, 1984.

Mahrle G, Hamme SM, Ippen H: Oral treatment of keratinizing disorders of skin and mucous membranes with etretinate. Arch Dermatol 118:97, 1982.

Mckie R: Current Perspectives in Immunodermatology. Churchill Livingstone, Edinburgh, 1984.

Melish ME, Hicks RM, Larson EJ: Mucocutaneous lymph node syndrome in the United States. Am J Dis Child 130:599, 1976.

Meyer JR, Migliorati CA, Daniels TE, Greenspan JS: Localization of basement membrane components in mucous membrane pemphigoid. J Invest Dermatol 84:105, 1985.

Milgrom H, Palmer EL, Slovin SF, et al: Kawasaki disease in a healthy young adult. Ann Intern Med 92:467, 1980.

Mobacken H, Nilsson LA, Olsson R, Sloberg K: Incidence of liver disease in chronic lichen planus of the mouth. Acta Derm Venereol (Stockh) 64:70, 1984.

Mostofi RS, Hayden NP, Soltani K: Oral malignant acanthosis nigricans. Oral Surg 56:372, 1983.

Moy W, Kumar V, Friedman RP, et al: Cicatricial pemphigoid: A case of onset at age 5. J Periodontol 57:39, 1986.

Moynahan EJ, Barnes PM: Zinc deficiency and a synthetic diet for lactose intolerance. Lancet 1:676, 1973.

Murti PK, Bhonsle RB, Deftany DC, Mehta FS: Oral lichen planus associated with pigmentation. J Oral Med 34:23, 1979.

Nazif MM, Ranalli DN: Stevens-Johnson syndrome: A report of fourteen cases. Oral Surg 53:263, 1982.

Newland JR, Leventon G: Warty dyskeratoma of the oral mucosa. Oral Surg 58:176, 1984.

Nisengard RJ, Chorzelski T, Maciejowska E, Kryst L: Dermatitis herpetiformis: IgA deposits in gingiva, buccal mucosa and skin. Oral Surg 54:22, 1982.

Olbricht SM, Flotte TJ, Collins AB, et al: Dermatitis herpetiformis. Cutaneous deposition of polyclonal IgA1. Arch Dermatol 122:418, 1986.

Röenick HH, Pearson RW: Epidermolysis bullosa acquisita. Arch Dermatol 117:383, 1981.

Rogers RS III, Van Hale HM: Immunopathologic diagnosis of oral mucosal inflammatory diseases. Australian J Dermatol 27:51, 1986.

Rosenbaum MM, Esterly NB, Creenwal MJ, Gerson CR: Cicatricial pemphigoid in a 6-year-old child: Report of a case and review of the literature. Pediatr Dermatol 2:13, 1984.

Sammarine MA, Loffredo A, Cecio A, et al: Stevens-Johnson syndrome: A clinical and histological study. Ophthalmologica 183:122, 1981.

Schiødt M, Permin H, Wilk A, et al: Oral lupus erythematosus, lichen planus and leukoplakia. An aid in diagnosis. Acta Pathol Microbiol Scand [C] 91:59, 1982.

Scully C, El-Kom M: Lichen planus: Review and update on pathogenesis. J Oral Pathol 14:431, 1985.

Sedano HO, Gorlin RJ: Acanthosis nigricans. Oral Surg 63:462, 1987.

Seghal VN: A clinical evaluation of 202 cases of vitiligo. Cutis 14:439, 1974.

Shklar G: Lichen planus as an oral ulcerative disease. Oral Surg 33:376, 1972.

Simon M, Djawari D, Schoenberger A: HLA antigens associated with lichen planus. Clin Exp Dermatol 9:435, 1984.

Sklavounou A, Laskaris G: Frequency of desquamative gingivitis in skin diseases. Oral Surg 56:141, 1983.

Tanay A, Mehregan AH: Warty dyskeratoma. Dermatologica 138:155, 1969.

Thomopoulou-Doukoudakis A, Squier C, Hill MW: Distribution of AB0 blood group substances in various types of oral lichen planus. J Oral Pathol 12:47, 1983.

Valaes T: Mucocutaneous lymph node syndrome in Athens, Greece. Pediatrics 55:295, 1975.

Watanabe T, Ohishi M, Tanaka K, Sato H: Analysis of HLA antigens in Japanese with oral lichen planus. J Oral Pathol 15:529, 1986.

Wells BT, Winkelmann RK: Acrodermatitis enteropathica: Report of 6 cases. Arch Dermatol 84:40, 1961.

Wojnarowska F, Marsden RA, Bhogal B, Black MM: Childhood cicatricial pemphigoid with linear IgA deposits. Clin Exp Dermatol 9:407, 1984.

Woodley DT, Briggaman RA, O'Keefe EJ, et al: Identification of the skin basement membrane autoantigen in epidermolysis bullosa acquisita. N Engl J Med 310:1007, 1984.

Wuepper KD, Watson PA, Kazmierowski JA: Immune complexes in erythema multiforme and the Stevens-Johnson syndrome. J Invest Dermatol 74:368, 1980.

Zegarelli DJ: Multimodality steroid therapy of erosive and ulcerative oral lichen planus. J Oral Med 38:127, 1983.

22. Hematologic Disorders

Alexander WN, Ferguson RL: Beta thalassemia minor and cleidocranial dysplasia: A rare combination of genetic abnormalities in one family. Oral Surg 49:413, 1980.

Baird IM, Dodge OG, Palmer FJ, Wawman RJ: The tongue and oesophagus in iron deficiency aneamia and effect of iron therapy. J Clin Pathol 14:603, 1961.

Berlin NJ: Diagnosis and classification of the polycythemias. Semin Hematol 12:339, 1976.

Beveridge BR, Bannerman RM, Evanson JM, Witts LJ: Hypochromic anaemia: A retrospective study and follow-up of 378 patients. Q J Med 34:145, 1965.

Drummond JF, White DK, Damm DD: Megaloblastic anemia with oral lesions: A consequence of gastric bypass surgery. Oral Surg 59:149, 1985.

Fotos PG, Graham WL, Bowers DC, Perfetto SP: Chronic autoimmune thrombocytopenic purpura. Oral Surg 56:564, 1983.

Goldfarb A, Nitzan DW, Marmary Y: Changes in the parotid salivary gland of β-thalassemia patients due to hemosiderin deposits. Int J Oral Surg 12:115, 1983.

Gorlin RJ, Chaudhry AP: The oral manifestations of cyclic (periodic) neutropenia. Arch Dermatol 82:344, 1960.

Greenberg MS: Clinical and histologic changes of the oral mucosa in pernicious anemia. Oral Surg 52:38, 1981.

Jacobs A, Cavill T: The oral lesions of iron deficiency anaemia. Pyridoxin and riboflavin status. Br J Haematol 14:291, 1968.

James WD, Guiry C, Grote W: Acute idiopathic thrombocytopenic purpura. Oral Surg 57:149, 1984.

Koller AZ: Immune thrombocytopenic purpura. Med Clin North Am 64:761, 1980.

Logothetis J, Economidou J, Costantoulakis M, et al: Cephalofacial deformities in thalassemia major (Cooley's anemia). Am J Dis Child 121:300, 1971.

Millard HD, Gobetti JP: Nonspecific stomatitis: A presenting sign in pernicious anemia. Oral Surg 39:562, 1975.

Ranasinghe AW, Warnakulasuriya KA, Tennekoon GE, et al: Oral mucosal changes in iron deficiency anemia in a Sri Lankan female population. Oral Surg 55:29, 1983.

Sickles EA, Greene WH, Wiernik PH: Clinical presentation of infection in granulocytopenic patients. Arch Intern Med 135:715, 1975.

Van Dis ML, Langlais RP: The thalassemias: Oral manifestations and complications. Oral Surg 62:229, 1986.

Weatherall DJ, Clegg JB: The Thalassemia Syndromes, 3rd ed. Blackwell Scientific, Oxford, 1981.

Wintrobe MM: Clinical Hematology, 8th ed., Lea & Febiger, Philadelphia, 1981.

Wood MM, Elwood PC: Symptoms of iron deficiency anaemia: A community survey. Br J Prev Soc Med 20:117, 1966.

23. Metabolic Diseases

Calkins E: Amyloidosis of the skin. In: Fitzpatrick T, Eisen AZ, Wolff K, et al (eds): Dermatology in General Medicine. Mc Graw Hill, New York, 1987, pp 1656–1657.

Chevrant-Breton J, Simon M, Bourel M, Ferrand B: Cutaneous manifestations of idiopathic hemochromatosis. Arch Dermatol 113:161, 1977.

Crosby WH: Hemochromatosis: the unsolved problems. Semin Hematol 14:135, 1977.

Dean DH, Hiramoto RN: Submandibular salivary gland involvement in hemochromatosis. J Oral Med 39:197, 1984.

Di Sant' Agnese PA, Davis PB: Cystic fibrosis in adults. Am J Med 66:121, 1979.

Finkelstein MW, Hammond HL, Jones RB: Hyalinosis cutis et mucosae. Oral Surg 54:49, 1982.

Franklin EC: Amyloid and amyloidosis of the skin. J Invest Dermatol 67:451, 1976.

Gilhuus-Moc O, Koppang H: Oral manifestations of porphyria. Oral Surg 33:926, 1972.

Goette DK, Carpenter WM: The mucocutaneous marker of pseudoxanthoma elasticum. Oral Surg 51:68, 1981.

Gorsky M, Silverman S, Lozada F, Kushner J: Histiocytosis-X: Occurrence and oral involvement in six adolescent and adult patients. Oral Surg 55:24, 1983.

Granda FM, Mc Daniel RK: Multiple progressive eosinophilic granuloma of the jaws. J Oral Maxillofac Surg 40:174, 1982.

Greenberger JS, Crocker AC, Vawter G, et al: Results of treatment of 127 patients with systemic histiocytosis (Letterer-Siwe syndrome, Schüller-Christian syndrome and multifocal eosinophilic granuloma). Medicine (Baltimore) 60:311, 1981.

Hansen RC, Lemen R, Revsin B: Cystic fibrosis manifesting with acrodermatitis enteropathica-like eruption. Arch Dermatol 119:51, 1983.

Harper JI, Duance VC, Sims TJ, Light ND: Lipoid proteinosis: An inherited disorder of collagen metabolism? Br J Dermatol 113:145, 1985.

Hartman KS: Histiocytosis-X: A review of 114 cases with oral involvement. Oral Surg 49:38, 1980.

Hofer P-A, Bergenholtz A: Oral manifestations in Urbach-Wiethe disease (lipoglycoproteinosis; lipoid proteinosis; hyalinosis cutis et mucosae). Odont Revy 26:39, 1975.

Kyle RA, Bayrd ED: Amyloidosis: Review of 236 cases. Medicine (Baltimore) 54:271, 1975.

Kyle RA: Amyloidosis. Part 2. Int J Dermatol 120:20, 1981.

Meenan FO, Bowe SD, Dinn JJ, et al: Lipoid proteinosis: A clinical, pathological and genetic study. Q J Med 47:549, 1978.

Moschella SL: Cutaneous xanthomatoses: A review and their relationship with the current classification of the hyperlipoproteinemias. Lahey Clin Found Bull 19:106, 1970.

Murphy GM, Hawk JLM, Nicholson DS, Magnus IA: Congenital erythropoitic porphyria (Günther's disease). Clin Exp Dermatol 12:61, 1987.

Rapidis AD, Langdon JD, Patel MF: Histiocytosis-X: Current concepts and a report of two cases. Br J Oral Surg 16:219, 1978.

Rye RJ: Porphyrias. In: Rook A, Wilkinson DS, Ebling FJG (eds): Textbook of Dermatology. Blackwell Scientific Publications, Oxford, 1986, pp 2271–2285.

Rayne J: Porphyria erythropoietica. Br J Oral Surg 5:68, 1967.

Rook A: Lipoid proteinosis: Urbach-Wiethe disease. Br J Dermatol 94:341, 1976.

Salisbury PL, Jacoway JR: Oral amyloidosis: A late complication of multiple myeloma. Oral Surg 56:48, 1983.

Schwartz HC, Olson DJ: Amyloidosis: A rational approach to diagnosis by intraoral biopsy. Oral Surg 39:837, 1975.

Shahani RT, Ward AM: Letterer-Siwe disease in a young adult. Br J Dermatol 89:313, 1973.

Stanbury JB, Wyngaarden JB, Fredrickson DS, et al: The Metabolic Basis of Inherited Diseases, 5th ed. McGraw-Hill, New York, 1983.

Tygstrup I, Haase E, Flensborg EW: The diagnostic value of lip biopsy in mucoviscoidosis. Acta Paediatr Scand 58:208, 1969.

Ward-Booth P, Ferguson MM, Mc Donald DG: Salivary gland involvement in hemochromatosis. Oral Surg 51:487, 1981.

Zuendel MT, Bowers DF, Kramer RN: Recurrent histiocytosis-X with mandibular lesions. Oral Surg 58:420, 1984.

24. Nutritional Disorders

Afonsky D: Stomatitis in nutritional deficiencies. Int Dent J 5:59, 1955.

Stratigos J, Katsambas A: Pellagra: A still existing disease. Br J Dermatol 96:99, 1977.

Stratigos J, Katsambas A: Pellagra: "Reappraisal." Acta Vitaminol Enzymol (Milano) 4:115, 1982.

Tillman HT: Oral and systemic changes in acute adult scurvy. Oral Surg 14:877, 1961.

25. Endocrine Diseases

Bartolocci EG, Parkes RB: Accelerated periodontal breakdown in uncontrolled diabetes. Oral Surg 52:387, 1981.

Bernick SM, Cohen DW, Baker L, Laster L: Dental disease in children with diabetes mellitus. J Periodontol 46:241, 1975.

Cohen WD, Friedman LA, Shapiro J, et al: Diabetes mellitus and periodontal disease: Two years longitudinal observations. Part I. J Periodontol 41:709, 1970.

Farman AG: Atrophic lesions of the tongue among diabetic outpatients: Their incidence and regression. J Oral Pathol 6:396, 1977.

Nerup J: Addison's disease – clinical studies: A report of 180 cases. Acta Endocrinol (Copenh) 76:127, 1974.

Russotto SB: Asymptomatic parotid gland enlargement in diabetes mellitus. Oral Surg 52:594, 1981.

Silverman S Jr, Ware WH, Gillooly C: Dental aspects of hyperparathyroidism. Oral Surg 26:184, 1968.

Warnakulasuriya S, Markwell RD, Williams DM: Familial hyperparathyroidism associated with cementifying fibromas of the jaws in two siblings. Oral Surg 59:269, 1985.

Wilson JB, Foster DW: William's Textbook of Endocrinology, 7th ed. W.B. Saunders, Philadelphia, 1985.

Wittmann AL: Macroglossia in acromegaly and hypothyroidism. Virchows Arch [A] 373:353, 1977.

26. Diseases of the Peripheral Nervous System

Bannister R: Brain's Clinical Neurology, 6th ed. Oxford University Press, Oxford, 1985.

Burzynski NJ, Weisskopf B: Familial occurrence of Bell's palsy. Oral Surg 36:504, 1973.

Dejong RN: The Neurologic Examination, 4th ed. Harper & Row, Philadelphia, 1979.

Hornstein OP: Melkersson-Rosenthal syndrome: A neuromucocutaneous disease of complex origin. Curr Probl Dermatol 5:117, 1973.

Kime CE: Bell's palsy: A new syndrome associated with treatment by nicotinic acid. Arch Otolaryngol 68:28, 1958.

Worsaae N, Pindborg JJ: Granulomatous gingival manifestations of Melkersson-Rosenthal syndrome. Oral Surg 49:131, 1980.

Worsaae N, Christensen KC, Schiødt M, Reibel J: Melkersson-Rosenthal syndrome and cheilitis granulomatosa. Oral Surg 54:404, 1982.

27. Precancerous Lesions

Bánóczy J: Follow-up studies in oral leukoplakia. J Maxillofac Surg 5:69, 1977.

Bánóczy J, Röed-Petersen B, Pindborg JJ, Inovay J: Clinical and histologic studies on electrogalvanically induced oral white lesions. Oral Surg 48:319, 1979.

Baric JM, Alman JE, Feldman RS, Chauncey HH: Influence of cigarette, pipe, and cigar smoking, removable partial dentures and age on oral leukoplakia. Oral Surg 54:424, 1982.

Bouquot JE, Gorlin RJ: Leukoplakia, lichen planus, and other oral keratoses in 23,616 white Americans over the age of 35 years. Oral Surg 61:373, 1986.

Bovopoulou O, Sklavounou A, Laskaris G: Loss of intercellular substance antigens in oral hyperkeratosis, epithelial dysplasia and squamous cell carcinoma. Oral Surg 60:648, 1985.

Cawson RA: Chronic oral candidiasis and leukoplakia. Oral Surg 22:582, 1966.

Cawson RA, Lehner T: Chronic hyperplastic candidiasis-candidal leukoplakia. Br J Dermatol 80:9, 1968.

Eyre J, Nally FF: Oral candidosis and carcinoma. Br J Dermatol 85:73, 1971.

Hong WK, Endicott J, Itri LM, et al: 13-Cis-retinoid acid in the treatment of oral leukoplakia. N Engl J Med 315:1501, 1986.

Greenspan D, Greenspan JS, Conant M, et al: Oral "hairy" leukoplakia in male homosexuals: Evidence of association with both papillomavirus and a herpes-group virus. Lancet 2:831, 1984.

Jones JH, Russel C: Candidal infection and leukoplakia. Br J Oral Surg 11:177, 1973.

Knapp MJ: Oral disease in 181,338 consecutive oral examinations. J Am Dent Assoc 83:1288, 1971.

Kramer IRH, El-Labban N, Lee KW: The clinical features and risk of malignant transformation in sublingual keratosis. Br Dent J 144:171, 1978.

Laskaris G, Nicolis G: Erythroplakia of Queyrat of the oral mucosa. Dermatologica, 162:395, 1981.

Mackenzie IC, Dabelsteen E, Squier CA: Oral Premalignancy. University of Iowa Press, Iowa City, 1980.

Mehta FS, Pindborg JJ, Cupta PC, Daftary DK: Epidemiologic and histologic study of oral cancer and leukoplakia among 50,915 villagers in India. Cancer 24:832, 1969.

Pindborg JJ: Oral Cancer and Precancer. John Wright and Sons, Bristol, 1980.

Reichart PA, Althoff J: Oral leukoplakia: A scanning electron microscopic study of epithelial surface patterns. Int J Oral Surg 12:159, 1983.

Shafer WG, Waldron CA: Erythroplakia of the oral cavity. Cancer 36:1021, 1975.

Silverman S Jr, Gorsky M, Lozada F: Oral leukoplakia and malignant transformation: A follow-up study of 257 patients. Cancer 53:563, 1984.

Silverman S Jr: Oral Cancer, 2nd ed. American Cancer Society, New York, 1985.

Waldron CA, Shafer WG: Leukoplakia revisited. A clinicopathologic study of 3256 oral leukoplakias. Cancer 36:1386, 1975.

WHO Collaborating Centre for Oral Precancerous Lesions: Definition of leukoplakia and related lesions: An aid to studies on oral precancer. Oral Surg 46:518, 1978.

28. Precancerous Conditions

Chierici G, Silverman S Jr, Forsythe B: A tumor registry study of oral squamous carcinoma. J Oral Med 23:91, 1968.

Fulling HJ: Cancer development in oral lichen planus. Arch Dermatol 108:667, 1973.

Holmstrup P, Pindborg JJ: Erythroplakia lesions in relation to oral lichen planus. Acta Derm Venereol [Suppl] (Stockh) 85:77, 1979.

Kraemer KH, Lee MM, Scotto J: Xeroderma pigmentosum: Cutaneous, ocular and neurologic abnormalities in 830 published cases. Arch Dermatol 123:241,1987.

Krutchkoff DJ, Cutler L, Laskowski S: Oral lichen planus: The evidence regarding potential malignant transformation. J Oral Pathol 7:1, 1978.

Larsson LG, Sandström A, Westling P: Relationship of Plummer-Vinson disease to cancer of the upper alimentary tract in Sweden. Cancer Res 35:3308,1975.

Laskaris G, Bovopoulou O, Nicolis G: Oral submucous fibrosis in a Greek female. Br J Oral Surg 19:197,1981.

Mackenzie IC, Dabelsteen E, Squier CA: Oral Premalignancy. University of Iowa Press, Iowa City,1980.

Mayer I, Abbey LM: The relationship of syphilis to primary carcinoma of the tongue. Oral Surg 30:678, 1970.

Murti PR, Daftary DK, Cupta PC, et al: Malignant potential of oral lichen planus: Observations in 72 patients from India. J Oral Pathol 15:71, 1986.

Pindborg JJ: Is submucous fibrosis a precancerous condition in the oral cavity? Int Dent J 22:474, 1972.

Pindborg JJ, Bhonsle RB, Murti PR,et al: Incidence and early forms of oral submucous fibrosis. Oral Surg 50:40, 1980.

Pogrel MA, Weldon LL: Carcinoma arising in erosive lichen planus in the midline of the dorsum of the tongue. Oral Surg 55:62, 1983.

Silverman S Jr, Griffith M: Studies on oral lichen planus. II. Follow-up on 200 patients, clinical characteristics and associated malignancy. Oral Surg 37:705, 1974.

Silverman S Jr: Oral Cancer, 2nd ed. American Cancer Society, New York, 1985.

Yagi KI, El-Casim A, Abbas KED, Prabhu SR: Carcinoma of the tongue in a patient with xeroderma pigmentosum. Int J Oral Surg 10:73, 1981.

Yagi KI, Prabhu SR: Carcinoma of the lip in xeroderma pigmentosum. J Oral Med 38:97, 1983.

Wynder EL, Bross IJ, Feldman RM: A study of the etiological factors in cancer of the mouth. Cancer 10:1300, 1957.

29. Malignant Neoplasms

Aberle AM, Abrams AM, Bowe R, et al: Lobular (polymorphous low-grade) carcinoma of minor salivary glands. Oral Surg 60:387, 1985.

Ackerman LV: Verrucous carcinoma of the oral cavity. Surgery 23:670, 1948.

Ajagbe HA, Daramola JO, Junaid TA: Chondrosarcoma of the jaws: Review of fourteen cases. J Oral Maxillofac Surg 43:763, 1985.

Batsakis JG, Pinkston GR, Byers RM, et al: Adenocarcinomas of the oral cavity: A clinicopathologic study of terminal duct carcinomas. J Laryngol Otol 97:825, 1983.

Brocheriou C, Crepy C, Guilbert F, et al: Tumeurs des glandes salivaires accessoires de la cavité buccale: Etude de 296 cas. Bull Cancer (Paris) 67:29, 1980.

Brodsky G, Rabson AB: Metastasis to the submandibular gland as the initial presentation of small cell ("oat cell") lung carcinoma. Oral Surg 58:76, 1984.

Carr RJ, Green DM: Oral presentation of disseminated angiosarcoma. Br J Oral Maxillofac Surg 24:277, 1986.

Chau MNY, Radden BG: Intra-oral salivary gland neoplasms: A retrospective study of 98 cases. J Oral Pathol 15:339, 1986.

Chaudhry AP, Hampel A, Gorlin RJ: Primary malignant melanoma of the oral cavity: A review of 105 cases. Cancer 11:923, 1958.

Chaudhry AP, Robinovitch MR, Mitchell DF: Chondrogenic tumors of the jaws. Am J Surg 102:403, 1961.

Chaudhry AP, Vickers RA, Gorlin RJ: Intraoral minor salivary gland tumors. Oral Surg 14:1194, 1961.

Chen KTK: Clear cell carcinoma of the salivary gland. Hum Pathol 14:91, 1983.

Clark WH Jr, From L, Bernardino E, Mihm MC: The histogenesis and biologic behavior of primary human malignant melanomas of the skin. Cancer Res 29:705, 1969.

Cooke BED: Recognition of oral cancer. Causes of delay. Br Dent J 142:96, 1977.

Dahlin DC, Unni KK: Osteosarcoma of bone and its important recognizable varieties. Am J Surg Pathol 1:61, 1977.

Douglass CW, Gammon MD: Reassessing the epidemiology of lip cancer. Oral Surg 57:631, 1984.

Eckardt A, Nommels R: Breast carcinoma metastatic to the gingiva. J Oral Maxillofac Surg 44:902, 1986.

Eisenberg E, Rosenberg B, Krutchkoff D: Verrucous carcinoma: A possible viral pathogenesis. Oral Surg 59:52, 1985.

Ellis GL, Corio RL: Spindle cell carcinoma of the oral cavity. Oral Surg 50:523, 1980.

Eneroth CM: Salivary gland tumors in the parotid gland, submandibular gland and the palate region. Cancer 27:1415, 1971.

Evans HL, Batsakis JG: Polymorphous low-grade adenocarcinomas of minor salivary glands: A study of fourteen cases of a distinctive neoplasm. Cancer 53:935, 1984.

Eversole LR, Leider AS, Jacobsen PL, Shaber EP: Oral Kaposi's sarcoma associated with acquired immunodeficiency syndrome among homosexual males. J Am Dent Assoc 107:248, 1983.

Eveson JW, Cawson RA: Tumours of the minor (oropharyngeal) salivary glands: A demographic study of 336 cases. J Oral Pathol 14:500, 1985.

Farman AG, Uys PB: Oral Kaposi's sarcoma. Oral Surg 39:288, 1975.

Forteza G, Colmenero B, López-Barea F: Osteogenic sarcoma of the maxilla and mandible. Oral Surg 62:179, 1986.

Gardner DG, Bell MA, Wesley RK, Wysocki GP: Acinic cell tumors of minor salivary glands. Oral Surg 50:545, 1980.

Hatziotis J, Constantinidis H, Papanayotou PH: Metastatic tumors of the oral soft tissues. Oral Surg 36:544, 1973.

Huvos AG, Rosen G, Dabska M, Marcove RC: Mesenchymal chondrosarcoma: A clinicopathologic analysis of 35 patients with emphasis on treatment. Cancer 51:1230, 1983.

Isaacson G, Shear M: Intraoral salivary gland tumors: A retrospective study of 201 cases. J Oral Pathol 12:57, 1983.

Jacoway JR, Nelson JF, Boyers RC: Adenoid squamous cell carcinoma (adenoacanthoma) of the oral labial mucosa. A clinicopathologic study of fifteen cases. Oral Surg 32:444, 1971.

Kato T, Takematsu H, Tomita Y, et al: Malignant melanoma of mucous membranes: A clinicopathologic study of 13 cases in Japanese patients. Arch Dermatol 123:216, 1987.

Kaugars GE, Svirsky JA: Lung malignancies metastatic to the oral cavity. Oral Surg 51:179, 1981.

La Riviere W, Pickett AB: Clinical criteria in diagnosis of early squamous cell carcinoma of the lower lip. J Am Dent Assoc 99:972, 1979.

Lindqvist C, Teppo L, Sane J, et al: Osteosarcoma of the mandible: Analysis of nine cases. J Oral Maxillofac Surg 44:759, 1986.

Lucas RB: Pathology of Tumor of the Oral Tissues, 4th ed. Churchill-Livingstone. Edinburgh, 1984.

Luna MA, Ordonez NG, Mackay B, et al: Salivary epithelial-myoepithelial carcinomas of intercalated ducts: A clinical, electron microscopic, and immunocytochemical study. Oral Surg 59:482, 1985.

Macht SD: Current concepts in melanoma. Otolaryngol Clin North Am 15:241, 1982.

Mackie RM: The immune response in human malignant melanoma. Clin Exp Dermatol 1:23, 1976.

Mc Coy JM, Waldron CA: Verrucous carcinoma of the oral cavity. Oral Surg 52:623, 1981.

Mc Govern VJ: The classification of melanoma and its relationship with prognosis. Pathology 2:85, 1970.

Mc Millan MD, Smillie AC, Ferguson JW: Malignant fibrous histiocytoma of the tongue: Report of a case and ultrastructural observations. J Oral Pathol 15:255, 1986.

Martis C: Chondrosarcoma of the mandible: Report of case. J Oral Surg 36:227, 1978.

Mashberg A, Meyers H: Anatomical site and size of 222 early asymptomatic oral squamous cell carcinomas. Cancer 37:2149, 1976.

Milton GW: Malignant Melanoma of the Skin and Mucous Membranes. Churchill-Livingstone, London, 1977.

Modlin RL, Hofman FM, Kempf R, et al: Kaposi's sarcoma in homosexual men: An immunohistochemical study. J Am Acad Dermatol 8:620, 1983.

Molnar L, Ronay P, Tapolcsanyi L: Carcinoma of the lip: Analysis of the material of 25 years. Oncology 29:101, 1974.

Neiders ME: Early clinical diagnosis of oral cancer. Int Dent J 22:441, 1972.

Nunnery EW, Kahn LB, Reddick RL, Lipper S: Hemangiopericytoma. Cancer 47:906, 1981.

O'Day RA, Soule EH, Gores RJ: Soft tissue sarcomas of the oral cavity. Mayo Clin Proc 39:169, 1964.

Ogus HD, Bennet MH: Carcinoma of the dorsum of the tongue: A rarity of misdiagnosis. Br J Oral Surg 16:115, 1978.

Oikarinen VJ, Calonius PE, Sainio P: Metastatic tumors to the oral region. I. An analysis of cases in the literature. Proc Finn Dent Soc 71:58, 1975.

Pindborg JJ: Oral Cancer and Precancer. John Wright and Sons, Bristol, 1980.

Pizer ME, Dubois DD: Adenoid cystic carcinoma of the upper lip. Oral Surg 59:70, 1985.

Saw D: Fibrosarcoma of maxilla. Oral Surg 47:164, 1979.

Sawyer DR, Nwoku AL, Kekere-Ekun AT: Chondrosarcoma of the jaws: Report of two cases. J Oral Med 42:30, 1987.

Scully C: Viruses and cancer: Herpes viruses and tumors in the head and neck. Oral Surg 56:285, 1983.

Seifert G, Rieb H, Donath K: Klassifikation der Tumoren der kleinen Speicheldrüsen. Pathohistologische Analyse von 160 Tumoren. Laryngol Rhinol Otol (Stuttg) 59:379, 1980.

Silverman S Jr: Oral Cancer, 2nd ed. American Cancer Society, New York, 1985.

Solomon MP, Sutton AL: Malignant fibrous histiocytoma of the soft tissues of the mandible. Oral Surg 35:653, 1973.

Spiro RH, Koss LG, Hajdu SI, Strong EW: Tumors of minor salivary origin. A clinicopathologic study of 492 cases. Cancer 31:117, 1973.

Spiro RH, Alfonso AE, Farr HW, et al: Cervical node metastasis from epidermoid carcinoma of the oral cavity and oropharynx. Am J Surg 128:562, 1974.

Tagagi M, Ishikawa G, Mori W: Primary malignant melanoma of the oral cavity in Japan with special reference to mucosal melanosis. Cancer 34:358, 1974.

Thackray AC, Lucas RB: Tumors of the major salivary glands. AFIP, 1974.

Thompson SH, Shear M: Fibrous histiocytomas of the oral and maxillofacial regions. J Oral Pathol 13:282, 1984.

Tomich CE, Hutton CE: Adenoid squamous cell carcinoma of the lip: Report of cases. J Oral Surg 30:592, 1972.

Triantafyllou A, Laskaris G: Clear cell adenocarcinoma of the oral cavity. Iatriki 43:331, 1983.

Tsianos E, Banis C, Stefanaki-Nikou S, Drosos A: Mandibular gingival metastasis from a rectal adenocarcinoma. J Oral Maxillofac Surg 43:133, 1985.

Van Hale HM, Handlers JP, Abrams AM, Strahs G: Malignant fibrous histiocytoma, myxoid variant metastatic to the oral cavity. Report of a case and review of the literature. Oral Surg 51:156, 1981.

Welch RD, Hirsch SA, Davis RG: Melanoma with metastasis to an apical periodontal cyst. Oral Surg 59:189, 1985.

Wesley RK, Mintz SM, Wertheimer FW: Primary malignant hemangioendothelioma of the gingiva. Oral Surg 39:103, 1975.

Williams HK, Edwards MB, Adekeye EO: Mesenchymal chondrosarcoma. Int J Oral Maxillofac Surg 16:119, 1987.

Zachariadis N, Papadakou A, Koundouris J, Constantinidis J, Angelopoulos A: Primary hemangioendotheliosarcoma of the mandible: Review of the literature and report of a case. J Oral Surg 38:288, 1980.

Ziegler JL, Lutzner MA, Conant MA: Kaposi's sarcoma (multiple idiopathic sarcoma). In: Fitzpatrick TB, Eisen AZ, Wolff K, et al (eds): Dermatology in General Medicine, 3rd ed. edited by McGraw-Hill, New York, 1987, p 1078.

30. Malignancies of the Hematopoietic and Lymphatic Tissues

Ambrus JL, Ambrus M: Burkitt's lymphoma. J Med 12:385, 1981.

Adatia AK: Significance of jaw lesions in Burkitt's lymphoma. Br Dent J 145:263, 1978.

Barrett AP: A long-term prospective clinical study of oral complications during conventional chemotherapy for acute leukemia. Oral Surg 63:313, 1987.

Bathard-Smith PJ, Coonar HS, Markus AF: Hodgkin's disease presenting intraorally. Br J Oral Surg 16:64, 1978–79.

Bennett JH, Shankar S: Gingival bleeding as the presenting feature of multiple myeloma. Br Dent J 157:101, 1984.

Block P, Delden L, Van der Waal I: Non-Hodgkin's lymphoma of the hard palate. Oral Surg 47:445, 1979.

Bressman E, Decter JA, Chasens AI, Sackler RS: Acute myeloblastic leukemia with oral manifestations. Oral Surg 54:401, 1982.

Burkitt DP: The discovery of Burkitt's lymphoma. Cancer 51:1777, 1983.

Curtis AB: Childhood leukemias: Initial oral manifestations. J Am Dent Assoc 81:159, 1971.

Damm DD, White DK, Cibull ML, et al: Mycosis fungoides: Initial diagnosis via palatal biopsy with discussion of diagnostic advantages of plastic embedding. Oral Surg 58:413, 1984.

De-Thé G, Geser A, Day NE: Epidemiological evidence for causal relationship between Epstein-Barr virus and Burkitt's lymphoma from Uganda prospective study. Nature 274:756, 1978.

Dolin S, Dewar JP: Extramedullary plasmacytoma. Am J Pathol 32:83, 1956.

Dreizen S, McCredie KB, Keating MJ, Luna MA: Malignant gingival and skin "infiltrates" in adult leukemia. Oral Surg 55:572, 1983.

Dreizen S, McCredie KB, Keating MJ: Chemotherapy associated oral hemorrhages in adults with acute leukemia. Oral Surg 57:494, 1984.

Edelson RL: Cutaneous T-cell lymphoma: Mycosis fungoides, Sézary syndrome and other variants. J Am Acad Dermatol 2:89, 1980.

Eisenbud L, Sciubba J, Mir R, Sachs SA: Oral presentations in non-Hodgkin's lymphoma: A review of thirty-one cases. Part I. Data analysis. Oral Surg 56:151, 1983.

Eisenbud L, Sciubba J, Mir R, Sachs SA: Oral presentations in non-Hodgkin's lymphoma: A review of thirty-one cases. Part II. Fourteen cases arising in bone. Oral Surg 57:272, 1984.

Eisenbud L, Mir R, Sciubba J, Sachs SA: Oral presentations in non-Hodgkin's lymphoma: A review of thirty-one cases. Part III. Six cases in children. Oral Surg 59:44, 1985.

Epstein JB, Voss NJS, Stevenson-Moore P: Maxillofacial manifestations of multiple myeloma. Oral Surg 57:267, 1984.

Forman GH, Wesson CM: Hodgkin's disease of the mandible. Br J Oral Surg 7:146, 1970.

Fucuda Y, Ishida T, Fujimoto M, et al: Malignant lymphoma of the oral cavity: Clinicopathologic analysis of 20 cases. J Oral Pathol 16:8, 1987.

Gamble JW, Driscoll EJ: Oral manifestation of macroglobulinemia of Waldenström. Oral Surg 13:104, 1960.

Haidar Z: A review of non-Hodgkin's lymphoma of the oral cavity 1950–1980. J Oral Med 41:197, 1986.

Hashimoto N, Kurihara K, Sakai H: Extramedullary plasmacytoma with crystal inclusions arising from the palatal tonsil. J Oral Pathol 12:309, 1983.

Kurihara K, Sakai H, Hashimoto N: Russel body-like inclusions in oral B-lymphomas. J Oral Pathol 13:640, 1984.

Laskaris G, Nicolis G, Capetanakis J: Mycosis fungoides with oral manifestations. Oral Surg 46:40, 1978.

Laskaris G, Papavasiliou S, Bovopoulou O, Nicolis G: Association of oral pemphigus with lymphocytic leukemia. Oral Surg 50:244, 1980.

Laskaris G, Triantafyllou A, Bazopoulou E: Solitary plasmacytoma of oral soft tissues: Report of a case and review of literature. Iatriki 39:452, 1981.

Lehrer S, Roswit B, Federman Q: The presentation of malignant lymphoma in the oral cavity and pharynx. Oral Surg 41:441, 1976.

Lennert K: Histopathology of Non-Hodgkin's Lymphomas. Springer-Verlag, Berlin, 1981.

Loh HS: A retrospective evaluation of 23 reported cases of solitary plasmacytoma of the mandible, with an additional case report. Br J Oral Maxillofac Surg 22:216, 1984.

Lynch MA, Ship II: Initial oral manifestations of leukemia. J Am Dent Assoc 75:932, 1967.

Matthews JB, Basu MK: Plasma cell lesions within the oral tissues: Immunoperoxidase staining of routinely fixed and processed tissue. Oral Surg 54:414, 1982.

Poole AG, Marchetta FC: Extramedullary plasmacytoma of the head and neck. Cancer 22:14, 1968.

Raubenheimer EJ, Dauth J, De Coning JP: Multiple myeloma presenting with extensive oral and perioral amyloidosis. Oral Surg 61:492, 1986.

Regezi JA, Zarbo RJ, Keren OF: Plasma cell lesions of the head and neck: Immunofluorescent determination of clonality from formalin-fixed, paraffin-embedded tissue. Oral Surg 56:616, 1983.

Rosenberg SA, Diamond HD, Jaslowitz B, Craver LF: Lymphosarcoma: A review of 1269 cases. Medicine (Baltimore) 40:31, 1961.

Sariban E, Donahue A, Magrath IT: Jaw involvement in American Burkitt's lymphoma. Cancer 53:1777, 1984.

Smith JL, Butler JJ: Skin involvement in Hodgkin's disease. Arch Dermatol 114:1832, 1978.

Stafford R, Sonis S, Lockhart P, Sonis A: Oral pathoses as diagnostic indicators in leukemia. Oral Surg 50:134, 1980.

Tabachnick TT, Levine B: Multiple myeloma involving the jaws and oral soft tissues. J Oral Surg 34:931, 1976.

Tomich CM, Shafer WG: Lymphoproliferative disease of the hard palate: Clinicopathologic entity. Oral Surg 39:754, 1975.

Ultmann JE, Moran EM: Clinical course and complications in Hodgkin's disease. Arch Intern Med 131:332, 1966.

Waldenström J: Macroglobulinemia. Adv Metab Disord 2:115, 1965.

Webb HE, Harrison EG, Masson JK, ReMine WH: Solitary extramedullary myeloma (plasmacytoma) of the upper part of respiratory tract and oropharynx. Cancer 15:1142, 1962.

White GE: Oral manifestations of leukemia in children. Oral Surg 29:420, 1970.

Wintrobe MM: Clinical Hematology, 8th ed. Lea & Febiger, Philadelphia, 1981.

Wong DS, Fuller LM, Butler JJ, Shullenberger CC: Extranodal non-Hodgkin's lymphoma of the head and neck. Am J Roentgenol Radium Ther Nucl Med 123:471, 1975.

Wright JM, Balciunas BA, Huus JH: Mycosis fungoides with oral manifestations. Oral Surg 51:24, 1981.

Yoshimura Y, Takada K, Kawai N, et al: Two cases of plasmacytoma in the oral cavity. Int J Oral Surg 5:82, 1976.

31. Benign Neoplasms

Abbey LM, Page DG, Sawyer DR: The clinical and histopathologic features of a series of 464 oral squamous cell papillomas. Oral Surg 49:419, 1980.

Baden E, Pierce M, Selman AJ, et al: Intra-oral papillary cystadenoma lymphomatosum. J Oral Surg 34:533, 1976.

Bayer RA, Hardman FG: Intra-oral surgical management of cystic hygroma. Br J Oral Surg 14:36, 1976.

Buchner A, Hansen LS: Melanotic macule of the oral mucosa. Oral Surg 48:244, 1979.

Buchner A, Hansen LS: Pigmented nevi of the oral mucosa: A clinicopathologic study of 32 new cases and review of 75 cases from the literature. Oral Surg 49:55, 1980.

Buchner A, Hansen LS: The histomorphologic spectrum of peripheral ossifying fibroma. Oral Surg 63:452, 1987.

Buchner A, Hansen LS: Pigmented nevi or the oral mucosa: A clinicopathologic study of 36 new cases and review of 155 cases from the literature. Oral Surg 63:566, 1987.

Chau MNY, Radden BG: Intra-oral salivary gland neoplasms: A retrospective study of 98 cases. J Oral Pathol 15:339, 1986.

Chen SY, Miller AS: Neurofibroma and schwannoma of the oral cavity. Oral Surg 47:522, 1979.

Chen SY, Fantasia JE, Miller AS: Myxoid lipoma of oral soft tissue. Oral Surg 57:300, 1984.

Cherrick HM, Dunlap CL, King OH: Leiomyomas of the oral cavity: Review of the literature and clinicopathologic study of seven new cases. Oral Surg 35:54, 1973.

Damm DD, Neville BW: Oral leiomyomas. Oral Surg 47:343, 1979.

Elzay RP, Dutz W: Myxomas of the paraoral-oral soft tissues. Oral Surg 45:246, 1978.

Eneroth CM, Blanck C, Jacobsson PÄ: Carcinoma in pleomorphic adenoma of the parotid gland. Acta Otolaryngol 66:477, 1968.

Enzinger FM, Weiss SW: Soft-Tissue Tumors. C.V. Mosby, St. Louis, 1983.

Epivatianos A, Trigonidis G, Papanayotou P: Vascular leiomyoma of the oral cavity. J Oral Maxillofac Surg 43:377, 1985.

Eveson JW, Cawson RA: Tumours of the minor (oropharyngeal) salivary glands: A demographic study of 336 cases. J Oral Pathol 14:500, 1985.

Epker BN, Henny FA: Intraoral sebaceous gland adenoma. Cancer 27:987, 1971.

Erlandson RA, Cardon CC, Higgins PJ: Histogenesis of benign pleomorphic adenoma (mixed tumor) of the major salivary glands: An ultrastructural and immunohistochemical study. Am J Surg Pathol 8:803, 1984.

Fantasia JE, Miller AS: Papillary cystadenoma lymphomatosum arising in minor salivary glands. Oral Surg 52:411, 1981.

Hatziotis J: Lipoma of the oral cavity. Oral Surg 36:511, 1971.

Helwing EB, Hackney VC: Syringadenoma papilliferum. Lesions with and without naevus sebaceous and basal cell carcinoma. Arch Dermatol 71:361, 1955.

Hidano A: Natural history of nevus of Ota. Arch Dermatol 95:187, 1967.

Hoffman S, Martinez MG: Fibrous histiocytomas of the oral mucosa. Oral Surg 52:277, 1981.

Houston GD: The giant cell fibroma. A review of 464 cases. Oral Surg 53:582, 1982.

Ide F, Umemura S: A microscopic focus of traumatic neuroma with intralesional glandular structures: An incidental finding. Oral Surg 57:68, 1984.

Isacsson G, Shear M: Intraoral salivary gland tumors: A retrospective study of 201 cases. J Oral Pathol 12:57, 1983.

Kerpel MA, Freedman PD, Lumerman H: The papillary cystadenoma of minor salivary gland origin. Oral Surg 46:820, 1978.

Laskaris G, Skouteris C, Angelopoulos A: Compound nevus of the oral mucosa. Iatriki 34:457, 1978.

Laskaris G, Patsakas A, Papadakou A, Angelopoulos A: Melanotic freckle of Hutchinson's of the oral mucosa. Mat Med Greca 6:211, 1978.

Laskaris G, Giannoulopoulos A, Kariaba E, Arsenopoulos A: Melanotic neuroectodermal tumor of infancy. Mat Med Greca 8:226, 1980.

Laskaris G, Economopoulou P, Nicolis G: Keratoacanthoma of the oral mucosa. Report of a case. Odontiatriki 13:151, 1980.

Lea PJ, Pawlowski A: Human melanocytic naevi. Acta Derm Venereol [Suppl] (Stockh) 127:5, 1986.

Levine J, Krutchkoff DJ, Eisenberg E: Monomorphic adenoma of minor salivary glands: A reappraisal and report of nine new cases. J Oral Surg 39:101, 1981.

Lovas GL, Wysocki GP, Daley TD: The oral blue nevus: Histogenetic implications of its ultrastructural features. Oral Surg 55:145, 1983.

Louridis O, Markopoulos A, Laskaris G: Junctional nevus of the oral mucosa. Report of a case. Odontostomatol Progr 24:195, 1970.

Luna MA, Stimson PG, Bardwill JM: Minor salivary gland tumors of the oral cavity. Oral Surg 25:71, 1968.

Martis C: Parotid benign tumors: Comments on surgical treatment of 263 cases. Int J Oral Surg 12:211, 1983.

Mc Coy JM, Mincer HH, Turner JE: Intraoral ancient neurilemoma (ancient schwannoma). Oral Surg 56:174, 1983.

Niizuma K: Syringocystadenoma papilliferum: Light and electron microscopic studies. Acta Derm Venereol (Stockh) 56:327, 1976.

Nowparast B, Howell FV, Rick GM: Verruciform xanthoma. Oral Surg 51:619, 1981.

Orlian A, Salman L, Reddi T, et al: Sebaceous adenoma of the oral mucosa. J Oral Med 42:38, 1987.

Papanicolaou S, Eversole LR: Glandular structures in neural sheath neoplasms. Oral Surg 53:69, 1982.

Papanicolaou S, Pierrakou E, Patsakas A: Intraoral blue nevus. J Oral Med 40:32, 1985.

Rapidis A: Lipoma of the oral cavity. Int J Oral Surg 11:30, 1982.

Rapidis A, Triantafyllou A: Myxoma of the oral soft tissue. J Oral Maxillofac Surg 41:188, 1983.

Seifert G, Rieb H, Donath K: Klassifikation der Tumoren der kleinen Speicheldrüsen. Pathohistologische Analyse von 160 Tumoren. Z. Laryngol Rhinol 59:379, 1980.

Seifert G, Miehlke A, Haubrich J, Chilla R: Diseases of the Salivary Glands. Georg Thieme Verlag, Stuttgart, 1986.

Shapiro L, Zegarelli DJ: The solitary labial lentigo: A clinicopathologic study of 20 cases. Oral Surg 31:87, 1971.

Sist TC, Greene GW: Traumatic neuroma of the oral cavity. Oral Surg 51:394, 1981.

Sklavounou A, Laskaris G, Angelopoulos A: Verruciform xanthoma of the oral mucosa. Dermatologica 164:41, 1982.

Thompson SH, Shear M: Fibrous histiocytomas of the oral and maxillofacial regions. J Oral Pathol 13:284, 1984.

Triantafyllou A, Sklavounou A, Laskaris G: Benign fibrous histiocytoma of the oral mucosa. J Oral Med 40:36, 1985.

Triantafyllou A, Laskaris G: Papillary syringadenoma of the lower lip: Report of a case. J Oral Maxillofac Surg 45:884, 1987.

Weathers DR, Callihan MD: Giant cell fibroma. Oral Surg 37:374, 1974.

Weathers DR, Corio RL, Grawford BE, et al: The labial melanotic macule. Oral Surg 42:196, 1976.

Wright BA, Jackson D: Neural tumors of the oral cavity. Oral Surg 49:509, 1980.

Zachariades N: Schwannoma of the oral cavity: Review of the literature and report of a case. J Oral Med 39:41, 1984.

32. Other Salivary Glands Disorders

Abrams AM, Melrose RJ, Howell FV: Necrotizing sialometaplasia: A disease simulating malignancy. Cancer 32:130, 1973.

Anneroth G, Hansen LS: Necrotizing sialometaplasia: The relationship of its pathogenesis to its clinical characteristics. Int J Oral Surg 11:283, 1982.

Bertram U: Xerostomia. Acta Odontol Scand (Suppl) 49:1, 1967.

Chaudhry AP, Yamane GM, Salman L, et al: Necrotizing sialometaplasia of palatal minor salivary glands: A report on 2 cases. J Oral Med 40:2, 1985.

Kinney RB, Burton CS, Vollmer RT: Necrotizing sialometaplasia: A sheep in Wolf's clothing. Arch Dermatol 122:208, 1986.

Lancaster JE, Hughes KW: Mikulicz's disease involving multiple salivary glands. Oral Surg 16:1266, 1963.

Mesa ML, Gertler RS, Schneider LC: Necrotizing sialometaplasia: Frequency of histologic misdiagnosis. Oral Surg 57:71, 1984.

Patton DW: Recurrent calculus formation following removal of the submandibular salivary gland. Br J Oral Maxillofac Surg 25:15, 1987.

Pullon PA, Miller AS: Sialolithiasis of accessory salivary glands: Review of 55 cases. J Oral Surg 30:832, 1972.

Rauch S: Die Speicheldrüsen des Menschen. Georg Thieme, Stuttgart, 1959.

Seifert G: Die pathologische Anatomie der Speicheldrüsenerkrankungen (Sialadenitis, Sialadenose, Sialome, Syndrome). HNO 13:1, 1965.

Seifert G, Miehlke A, Haubrich J, Chilla R: Diseases of the Salivary Glands. Georg Thieme Verlag, Stuttgart, 1986.

33. Tumorlike Lesions

Angelopoulos AP: Pyogenic granuloma of the oral cavity: Statistical analysis of its clinical features. J Oral Surg 29:840, 1971.

Apisarnthanarax P: Granular cell tumor. An analysis of 16 cases and review of the literature. J Am Acad Dermatol 5:171, 1981.

Darski K, Stoll HL Jr: Cutaneous horn arising in chronic discoid lupus erythematosus. Arch Dermatol 121:837, 1985.

De la Monte SM, Radowsky M, Hood AF: Congenital granular-cell neoplasms: An unusual case report with ultrastructural findings and a review of the literature. Am J Dermatopathol 8:57, 1986.

Fuhr AA, Krogh PHJ: Congenital epulis in the newborn. J Oral Surg 26:61, 1972.

Giansanti JS, Waldron CA: Peripheral giant cell granuloma: Review of 720 cases. J Oral Surg 27:787, 1969.

Henefer EP, Abaza NA, Anderson SP: Congenital granular-cell epulis. Oral Surg 47:515, 1979.

Lack EE, Worsham GF, Callihan MD, et al: Gingival granular cell tumors of the newborn (congenital "epulis"). A clinical and pathology study of 21 patients. Am J Surg Pathol 5:37, 1981.

Lifshitz MS, Flotte TJ, Greco MA: Congenital granular cell epulis. Immunohistochemical and ultrastructural observations. Cancer 53:1845, 1984.

Reis LT, Perini MO, Do Rosario M, et al: Cutaneous horn on the glans. Int J Dermatol 17:410, 1978.

Rohrer MD, Young SK: Congenital epulis (gingival granular cell tumor): Ultrastructural evidence of origin from pericytes. Oral Surg 53:56, 1982.

Samant A, Malick CP, Chabra S, et al: Gingivitis and periodontal disease in pregnancy. J Periodontol 47:419, 1976.

Schwartz RA, Stoll HL Jr: Cutaneous horn. In: Fitzpatrick TB, Eisen AZ, Wolff K, et al (eds): Dermatology in General Medicine, 3rd ed. Mc Graw-Hill, 1987, p 736.

Vilmann A, Vilmann P, Vilmann H: Pyogenic granuloma: Evaluation of oral conditions. Br J Oral Maxillofac Surg 24:376, 1986.

Welbury RR: Congenital epulis of the newborn. Br J Oral Surg 18:238, 1980.

Index

Numbers in **boldface** indicate pages with figures.

A

Abscess, oral soft tissue, 120, **121**
– periodontal, 76, **77**
Acanthosis nigricans benign, 18, **19**
– – malignant, 190, **191**
Acinic cell tumor, 238, **239**
Acquired Immune Deficiency Syndrome (AIDS), 112, **112–116**
Acrodermatitis enteropathica, 190, **191**
Actinic cheilitis, 88, **89**
Actinomycosis, 136, **137**
Acuminatum, condyloma, 108, **109**
Adenocarcinoma, 242, **243**
– clear cell, 242, **243**
Adenoid cystic carcinoma, 240, **241**
– squamous cell carcinoma, 236, **237**
Adenoma, pleomorphic, 288, **289**
– – malignant, 240, **241**
– sebaceous, 278, **279**
Adrenocortical insufficiency, 212, **213**
Agranulocytosis, 196, **197–199**
Alba, linea, 2, **3**
Alcohol burn, 52, **53**
Allergic stomatitis, acrylic resin, 72, **73**
– – eugenol, 72, **73**
Allergy to chemical agents applied locally, 72–73
Amalgam tattoo, 68, **69**
Amyloidosis, 202, **201, 202**
Anatomic variants, normal, 2, **3**
Anemia, aplastic, 198, **199**
– iron deficiency, 194, **195**
– pernicious, 194, **195**
Angioneurotic edema, 64, **65**
Angular cheilitis, 88, **89**
Ankyloglossia, 4, **5**
Anomalies, developmental, 4–11
Antibiotic-induced stomatitis, 60, **61**
Aphthous ulcers, major, 150, **151**
– – minor, 149, **149**
– – recurrent, 149
Aplastic anemia, 198, **199**
Ariboflavinosis, 209, **211**
Aspirin burn, 52, **52**
Atrophic candidosis, acute, 138, **139**
– – chronic, 138, **139**
– glossitis, 128, **129**
– – in tertialy syphilis, 226, **227**
Atrophy of the maxillary alveolar ridge, 46, **47**
Autoimmune diseases, 159–166
Azathioprine ulceration, 62, **63**

B

Bacterial infections, 117–137
Basal cell carcinoma, 238, **239**
Behçet's syndrome, 152, **152–154**
Benign acanthosis nigricans, 18, **19**
– fibrous histiocytoma, 274, **275**
– lymphoepithelial lesion, 164, **165**
– pemphigus, familial, 20, **21**
– tumors, 264–289
Bifid tongue, 6, **7**
– uvula, 6, **7**
Biliary cirrhosis, primary, 164, **165**
Bismuth deposition, 68, **69**
Biting, chronic, 40, **41**
Blastomycosis, North American, 144, **145**
Blue nevus, 284, **285**
Breathing, mouth and gingivitis, 76, **77**
Buccal cellulitis, 122, **123**
Bullosa, epidermolysis, 22, **23**
– – acquisita, 182, **183**
Burkitt's lymphoma, 258, **259**
Burn, acrylic resin, 52, **53**
– alcohol, 52, **53**
– aspirin, 52, **52**
– eugenol, 50, **51**
– iodine, 52
– paraformaldehyde, 54, **55**
– phenol, 50, **51**
– silver nitrate, 54, **55**
– sodium hypochlorite, 54, **55**
– – perborate, 54, **54**
– thermal, 58, **59**
– trichloroacetic acid, 50, **51**

C

Cancrum oris, 118, **119**
Candida-Endocrinopathy syndrome, 142, **143**
Candidal leukoplakia, 138, 224, **225**
Candidosis, 138
– atrophic, acute, 138, **139**
– chronic, hyperplastic, 138, **140**
– mucocutaneous, 142, **142, 143**
– multifocal, 140, **141**
– pseudomembranous, acute (thrush), 138, **139**
Carcinoma, adenoid cystic, 240, **241**
– adenoid squamous cell, 236, **237**
– basal cell, 238, **239**
– lymphoepithelial, 236, **237**
– minor salivary glands, lobular, 242, **243**
– spindle cell, 236, **237**
– squamous cell, 230, **231–234**
– verrucous, 234, **235, 236**
Cellulitis, buccal, 122, **123**
Chancroid, 130, **131**
Cheilitis, actinic, 88, **89**
– angular, 88, **89**
– contact, 90, **91**
– exfoliative, 88, **89**
– glandularis, 90, **91**
– granulomatosa, 90, **91**
– plasma cell, 92, **92**
– retinoids, 66, **67**
Chemical agents applied locally, allergy, 72–73
– – oral lesions, 50–55
Chondroectodermal dysplasia, 24, **25**
Chondrosarcoma, 248, **249**
Cirrhosis, biliary primary, 164, **165**
Cicatricial pemphigoid, 176, **177–179**
– – childhood, 178, **179**
Cigarette smoker's lip lesion, 58, **59**
Circumvallate papillae, hypertrophy, 86, **87**
Clear cell adenocarcinoma, 242, **243**
Cleft lip, 6, **6**
– palate, 6, **7**
Compound nevus, 282, **283**
Condyloma acuminatum, 108, **109**
Condylomata lata, 128, **128**
Conditions, precancerous, 226–229
Congenita, dyskeratosis, 14, **15**
– pachyonychia, 14, **14, 15**
Congenital syphilis, 130, **131**
– epulis of the newborn, 296, **297**
Contagiosum, molluscum, 110, **111**
Cotton roll stomatitis, 42, **43**
Cowden's disease, 30, **31**
Crenated tongue, 84, **85**
Crohn's disease, 158, **158**
Cunnilingus, lingual frenum ulcer, 42, **43**
Cutaneous horn, 280, **280, 281**
– leishmaniasis, 146, **147**
Cyclosporine, fibrous gingival hyperplasia, 64, **65**
Cystadenoma, papillary lymphomatosum, 288, **289**
Cyst, dermoid, 96, **96**

– eruption, 96, **97**
– gingival of the adult, 98, **99**
– – of the newborn, 96, **97**
– lymphoepithelial, 94, **95**
– mucocele, 93, **93, 94**
– palatine papilla, 98, **99**
– ranula, 94, **95**
– thyroglossal duct, 98, **99**
Cysts, soft tissue, 93–99
Cystic carcinoma, adenoid, 240, **241**
– fibrosis, 206, **206**
– hygroma, 278, **279**

D

Deficiency, iron, anemia, 194, **195**
– protein, 210, **211**
Denture stomatitis, 44, **45**
Deposition bismuth, 68, **69**
Deposits, metal and other, 68–69
Dermatitis herpetiformis, 182, **183**
– perioral, 192, **193**
Dermatomyositis, 162, **163**
Dermoid cyst, 96, **96**
Developmental anomalies, 4–11
– malformation, fibrous, 10, **10**
Diabetes mellitus, 212, **213**
Drugs oral lesions, 60–67
Dyskeratoma, warty, 192, **193**
Dyskeratosis, congenita, 14, **15**
– follicularis, 20, **20, 21**
– hereditary benign intraepithelial, 12, **13**
Dysplasia, cleidocranial, 32, **33**
– chondroectodermal, 24, **25**
– hypohidrotic ectodermal, 16, **16, 17**

E

Ectodermal dysplasia, hypohidrotic, 16, **16, 17**
Edema, angioneurotic, 64, **65**
Ehlers-Danlos syndrome, 36, **37**
Endocrine diseases, 212–215
Eosinophilic ulcer, 48, **49**
Epidermolysis bullosa, 22, **23**
– – acquisita, 182, **183**
Epulis fissuratum, 44, **45**
– of the newborn, congenital, 296, **297**
Erosions, palatal due to smoking, 56, **57**
Eruption cyst, 96, **97**
Erysipelas, 120, **121**
Erythema multiforme, 167, **167, 168**
Erythroleukemia, 256, **257**
Erythroplasia, 224, **225**
Exostoses, multiple, 8, **9**

F

Facial nerve, paralysis peripheral, 216, **217**
Factitious trauma, 40, **41**
Fellatio, 42, **43**
Fibroma, 266, **267**
– giant cell, 268, **268**
– – peripheral ossifying, 268, **269**
Fibromatosis, gingiva, 12, **13**
Fibrosarcoma, 244, **245**
Fibrosis, cystic, 206, **206**
– submucous, 226, **227**, **228**
Fibrous gingival hyperplasia due to phenytoin, 64, **65**
– histiocytoma, benign, 274, **275**
– – malignant, 246, **247**
Fissured tongue, 82, **83**
Fistula, granuloma, 294, **295**
– periodontal, 76, **77**
Focal dermal hypoplasia, 34, **35**
– epithelial hyperplasia, 110, **111**
Foliaceus, pemphigus, 174, **175**
Fordyce's granules, 4, **5**
Freckles, 280, **281**
Fungal infections, 138–145
Fungiform papillae hypertrophy, 86, **87**

G

Genetic diseases, 12–37
Geographic stomatitis, 80, **81**
– tongue, 80, **81**
Giant cell, fibroma, 268, **268**
– – granuloma, peripheral, 296, **296**, **297**
Gingiva, attached material alba, 68, **69**
Gingival cyst of the adult, 98, **99**
– – newborn, 96, **97**
– fibromatosis, 12, **13**
– fibrous hyperplasia due to phenytoin, 64, **65**
Gingivitis, 74, **75**
– acute necrotizing ulcerative, 117, **117**
– desquamative, 78, **79**
– and mouth breathing, 76, **77**
– plasma cell, 78, **79**
Gingivostomatitis, herpetic, primary, 100, **101**
– streptococcal, 118, **119**
Glandularis, cheilitis, 90, **91**
Glossitis, atrophic, 128, **129**
– – in tertiary syphilis, 226, **227**
– interstitial, 128, **129**
– plasma cell, 84, **85**
– rhomboid, median, 80, **81**
Glossodynia, 84, **85**
Gold-induced stomatitis, 60, **61**
Granular, cell tumor, 274, **274**
Granuloma, fistula, 294, **295**
– giant cell, peripheral, 296, **296**, **297**
– midline, lethal, 156, **157**
– postextraction, 294, **295**
– pregnancy, 293, **295**

– pyogenic, 293, **293**, **294**
Granulomatosa, cheilitis, 90, **91**
Granulomatosis Wegener's, 156, **157**
Gumma, 128, **129**

H

Hairy tongue, 82, **83**
Hand-foot-and-mouth disease, 106, **106**, **107**
Heerfordt's syndrome, 148, **148**
Hemangioma, 274, **275**, **276**
Hemangioendothelioma, 246, **247**
Hemangiopericytoma, 246, **247**
Hematoma, traumatic, 40, **40**
Hematologic disorders, 194–199
Hematopoietic and lymphatic tissues, malignancies, 252–263
Hemiatrophy, facial, 10, **11**
Hemorrhagic telangiectasia, hereditary, 26, **27**
Hemochromatosis, 204, **205**
Hepatitis, lupoid, 166, **166**
Hereditary dyskeratosis, intraepithelial benign, 12, **13**
Herpangina, 104, **105**
Herpes labialis, 102, **103**
– zoster, 102, **103**
Herpetic, gingivostomatitis primary, 100, **101**
– stomatitis, secondary, 100, **101**
Herpetiform ulcers, 150, **151**
Herpetiformis, dermatitis, 182, **183**
Histiocytoma fibrous, benign, 274, **275**
– – malignant, 246, **247**
Histiocytosis X, 206, **207**, **208**
Histoplasmosis, 144, **145**
Hodgkin's disease, 256, **257**, **258**
Hormone, sex disorders, 214, **215**
Horn, cutaneous, 280, **280**
– mucosal, 280, **281**
Hygroma, cystic, 278, **279**
Hyperparathyroidism, primary, 214, **215**
Hyperplasia, focal epithelial, 110, **111**
– fibrous gingival due to cyclosporine, 64, **65**
– – phenytoin, 64, **65**
Hyperplasia, papillary, palate, 44, **45**, 140, **141**
– due to negative pressure, 46, **47**
– verrucous, 264, **265**
Hyperplastic candidosis, chronic, 138, **140**
Hypertrophy, circumvallate papillae, 86, **87**
– foliate papillae, 86, **86**
– fungiform papillae, 86, **87**
– masseteric, 10, **11**
Hypoglossal nerve paralysis, 216, **217**
Hypoplasia, focal dermal, 34, **35**
Hypothyroidism, 212, **213**

I

Immunoglobulin A disease, linear, 180, **181**
Immunopathogenesis, diseases, 149–158
Incontinentia pigmenti, 34, **35**, **37**
Infections, bacterial, 117–137
– fungal, 138–145
– others, 146–148
– viral, 100–116
Injection, palatal necrosis, 48, **49**
Injuries, mechanical, 38–49
– radiation-induced, 70–71
Insufficiency, adrenocortical, 212, **213**
Interstitial glossitis, 128, **129**
Intramucosal nevus, 282, **283**
Iodine burn, 52, **53**
Iron deficiency anemia, 194, **195**

J

Junctional, nevus, 282, **283**
Juvenile, pemphigus vulgaris, 176, **176**
– periodontitis, 74, **75**

K

Kaposi's sarcoma, 244, **245**, **115**, **116**
Keratoacanthoma, 266, **267**
Klippel-Trenaunay-Weber syndrome, 30, **30**

L

Lata, condylomata, 128, **128**
Late syphilis, 128
Leiomyoma, 272, **273**
Leishmaniasis, cutaneous, 146, **147**
Lentigo, maligna, 286, **287**
– simplex, 280, **281**
Leprosy, 134, **135**
Lesion, lip in cigarette smokers, 58, **59**
– – lymphoepithelial, benign, 164, **165**
Lesions, oral, chemical agents, 50–55
– – drugs, 60–67
– – heat, 56–59
– – penicillamine-induced, 62, **63**
– precancerous, 219–225
– – tumor like, 293–297
Leukemias, 252
– acute, 252, **253**, **254**
– chronic, 254, **255**
Leukoedema, 2, **3**
Leukoplakia, 219, **219–225**
– candidal, 224, **225**
Lethal midline granuloma, 156, **157**
Lichen planus, 184, 228, **184–187**, **221**
Linea alba, 2, **3**
Lingual frenum ulcer, after cunnilingus, 42, **43**

Lip, double, 8, **8**
– cleft, 6, **6**
– pits, congenital, 4, **5**
Lipoid proteinosis, 202, **203**
Lips, diseases, 88–92
Lipoma, 268, **269**
Lobular carcinoma of minor salivary glands, 242, **243**
Lupoid hepatitis, 166, **166**
Lupus vulgaris, 134, **135**
– erythematosus, discoid, 159, **159**, **160**
– – systemic, 160, **161**
Lymph node, mucocutaneous syndrome, 188, **189**
Lymphangioma, 276, **277**
Lymphatic and hematopoietic tissues, malignancies, 252–263
Lymphoepithelial carcinoma, 236, **237**
– cyst, 94, **95**
– lesion, benign, 164, **165**
Lymphoma, Burkitt, 258, **259**
Lymphomas, non-Hodgkin's, 258, **259**
Lymphonodular pharyngitis, acute, 104, **105**

M

Macroglobulinemia, 260, **261**
Macular syphilides, 124, **125**
Maffucci's syndrome, 26, **27**
Major aphthous ulcers, 150, **151**
Malformation, developmental fibrous, 10, **10**
Malignancies of the hematopoietic and lymphatic tissues, 252–263
Malignant acanthosis nigricans, 190, **191**
– fibrous histiocytoma, 246, **247**
– melanoma, 248, **249**
– neoplasms, 230–251
– pleomorphic adenoma, 240, **241**
Mandibularis, torus, 8, **9**
Masseteric hypertrophy, 10, **11**
Material alba of the attached gingiva, 68, **69**
Maxillary alveolar ridge, atrophy, 46, **47**
Measles, 106, **107**
Mechanical injuries, 38–49
Median rhomboid glossitis, 80, **81**
Melanoma, malignant, 248, **249**
Melanotic neuroectodermal tumor of infancy, 286, **287**
Melkersson-Rosenthal syndrome, 218, **218**
Medicamentosa, stomatitis, 60, **61**
Metal and other deposits, 68–69
Metastatic tumors, 250, **250**, **251**
Methotrexate ulcerations, 62, **63**
Midline granuloma, lethal, 156, **157**
Mikulicz's syndrome, 290, **291**
Minor aphthous ulcers, 149, **149**
Molluscum contagiosum, 110, **111**
Mononucleosis, infectious, 108, **109**
Mucocele, 93, **93**, **94**
Mucocutaneous candidosis, chronic, 142, **142**, **143**
– lymph node syndrome, 188, **189**
Mucoepidermoid tumor, 240, **241**

Mucous patches, 124, **126**, **127**
Multifocal candidosis, chronic, 140, **141**
Multiple exostoses, 8, **9**
Mycosis fungoides, 260, **261**
Myeloma, multiple, 262, **263**
Myxoma, 270, **271**

N

Necrolysis, toxic epidermal, 170, **171**
Necrosis, palatal due to injection, 48, **49**
Necrotizing sialometaplasia, 290, **291**
– ulcerative gingivitis, acute, 117, **117**
– – stomatitis, acute, 118, **118**
Neoplasms, malignant, 230–251
Neurofibroma, 270, **271**
Neurofibromatosis, 24, **25**
Neuroma, traumatic, 272, **273**
Neutropenia, cyclic, 196, **197**
Nevus, blue, 284, **285**
– compound, 282, **283**
– intramucosal, 282, **283**
– junctional, 282, **283**
– Ota, 284, **285**
– white spongue, 12, **13**
Nicotinic stomatitis, 56, **56**, **57**
Nigricans, acanthosis, malignant, 190, **191**
– – benign, 18, **19**
Nitrate silver, burn, 54, **55**
Normal oral pigmentation, 2, **3**
Nutritional disorders, 209–211

O

Oral lesions due to chemical agents, 50–55
– – to drugs, 60–67
– – to heat, 56–59
– – penicillamine-induced, 62, **63**
– mucosa, plasmatocytoma, 262, **263**
– soft tissue abscess, 120, **121**
Oro-facial digital syndrome, 32, **33**
Osteosarcoma, 248, **250**
Ota, nevus, 284, **285**

P

Pachyonychia congenita, 14, **14**, **15**
Palatal erosions due to smoking, 56, **57**
– necrosis due to injection, 48, **49**
Palate, cleft, 6, **7**
Palatine papilla cyst, 98, **99**
Palatinus, torus, 8, **9**
Papillae circumvallate, hypertrophy, 86, **87**
– foliate, hypertrophy, 86, **87**
– fungiform, hypertrophy, 86, **87**
Papillary cystadenoma lymphomatosum, 288, **289**
– hyperplasia of the palate, 44, **45**, 140, **141**

– syringadenoma of the lower lip, 278, **279**
Papilloma, 264, **265**
Papillon-Lefèvre syndrome, 18, **19**
Papular syphilides, 126, **127**
Paralysis, hypoglossal nerve, 216, **217**
– peripheral facial nerve, 216, **217**
Parotitis, suppurative, acute, 122, **123**
Patches, mucous, 124, **126**, **127**
Pellagra, 209, **209**, **210**
Peutz-Jeghers syndrome, 26, **27**
Pemphigoid, bullous, 180, **181**
– cicatricial, 176, **177–179**
– – of childhood, 178, **179**
Pemphigus, 172
– erythematosus, 174, **175**
– familial, benign, 20, **21**
– foliaceus, 174, **175**
– vegetans, 174, **174**
– vulgaris, 172, **173**
– – juvenile, 176, **176**
Penicillamin-induced oral lesions, 62, **63**
Perborate sodium, burn, 54, **54**
Periodontal abscess, 76, **77**
– diseases, 74–79
– fistula, 76, **77**
Periodontitis, 74, **75**
– juvenile, 74, **75**
Perioral dermatitis, 192, **193**
Peripheral facial nerve paralysis, 216, **216**
– giant cell granuloma, 296, **296**, **297**
– nervous system, diseases, 216–-218
– ossifying fibroma, 268, **269**
Pernicious anemia, 194, **195**
Pharyngitis, lymphonodular acute, 104, **105**
Phenol burn, 50, **51**
Phenytoin, fibrous gingival hyperplasia, 64, **65**
Pigmentation due to antimalarials, 66, **67**
– oral, normal, 2, **3**
Pigmenti, incontinentia, 34, **35**, **37**
Pigmentosum, xeroderma, 228, **229**
Planus, lichen, 184, 228, **184–187**, **229**
Plasma cell cheilitis, 92, **92**
– – gingivitis, 78, **79**
– – glossitis, 84, **85**
Plasmatocytoma of the oral mucosa, 262, **263**
Pleomorphic adenoma, 288, **289**
– – malignant, 240, **241**
Plummer-Vinson syndrome, 194, 226, **195**, **227**
Polycythemia vera, 256, **257**
Porphyrias, 204, **205**
Postextraction granuloma, 294, **295**
Precancerous conditions, 226–229
– lesions, 219–225
Pregnancy granuloma, 293, **295**
Primary herpetic gingivostomatitis, 100, **101**
– hyperparathyroidism, 214, **215**
– syphilis, 124, **125**
Protein deficiency, 210, **211**
Pseudomembranous candidosis (thrush), acute, 138, **139**

Psoriasis, 188, **189**
Purpura, thrombocytopenic, 198, **199**
Pyogenic granuloma, 293, **293, 294**

R

Radiation-induced injuries, 70–71, **71**
Ranula, 94, **95**
Recurrent aphthous ulcers, 149
Reiter's syndrome, 154, **155**
Retinoids, cheilitis, 66, **67**
Rhomboid glossitis, median, 80, **81**

S

Salivary glands, carcinoma lobular of minor, 242, **243**
– – disorders, other, 290–292
Sarcoma Kaposi, 244, **245**
Sarcoidosis, 146, **147**
Scarlet fever, 120, **121**
Schwannoma, 270, **271**
Scleroderma, 160, **161–163**
Sclerosis, tuberous, 28, **28, 29**
Scurvy, 210, **211**
Sebaceous adenoma, 278, **279**
Secondary syphilis, 124
Sex hormone disorders, 214, **215**
Sialadenitis, acute submandibular, 122, **123**
Sialometaplasia, necrotizing, 290, **291**
Sialolithiasis, 290, **291**
Sjögren's syndrome, 164, **165**
Skin diseases, 167–193
Smoking, palatal erosions, 56, **56, 57**
Sodium hypochlorite burn, 54, **55**
– perborate burn, 54, **54**
Soft tissue cysts, 93–99
Spindle cell carcinoma, 236, **237**
Squamous cell carcinoma, 230, **231–234**
– – – adenoid, 236, **237**
Stevens-Johnson syndrome, 168, **169**
Stomatitis, allergic, due to acrylin resin, 72, **73**
– – eugenol, 72, **73**
– antibiotic-induced, 60, **61**
– cotton roll, 42, **43**
– denture, 44, **45**
– geographic, 80, **82**
– gold-induced, 60, **61**
– gonococcal, 130, **131**
– herpetic, secondary, 100, **101**
– medicamentosa, 60, **61**
– necrotizing, ulcerative, acute, 118, **118**
– nicotinic, 56, **56, 57**
Sturge-Weber syndrome, 28, **29**
Streptococcal gingivostomatitis, 118, **119**
Sublingual varices, 86, **87**
Suppurative parotitis, acute, 122, **123**
Syndrome
– Acquired immune deficieny, 112, **112–116**

– Behçet, 152, **152–154**
– Burneville-Pringle, 28, **28, 29**
– Candica-endocrinopathy, 142, **143**
– Ehlers-Danlos, 36, **37**
– Ellis-van Creveld, 24, **25**
– Goltz, 34, **35**
– Heerfordt, 148, **148**
– Focal palmoplantar and oral mucosa hyperkeratosis, 16, **17, 18**
– Jadassohn-Lewandowsky, 14, **14, 15**
– Klippel-Trenaunay-Weber, 30, **30, 31**
– Maffucci, 26, **27**
– Melkersson-Rosenthal, 218, **218**
– Mikulicz, 290, **291**
– Mucocutaneous lymph node, 188, **189**
– Oro-facial digital, 32, **33**
– Papillon-Lefèvre, 18, **19**
– Peutz-Jeghers, 26, **27**
– Plummer-Vinson, 194, 226, **195, 227**
– Reiter, 154, **155**
– Sjögren, 164, **165**
– Stevens-Johnson, 168, **169**
– Sturge-Weber, 28, **29**
– Zinsser-Engman-Cole, 14, **15**
Syphilis, 124
– congenital, 130, **131**
– late, 128
– primary, 124, **125**
– secondary, 124
– tertiary, glossitis atrophic, 226, **227**
Syphilides, macular, 124, **125**
– papular, 126, **127**
Syringadenoma, papillary of the lower lip, 278, **279**
Systemic lupus erythematosus, 160, **161**

T

Tattoo, amalgam, 68, **69**
Telangiectasia, hereditary hemorrhagic, 26, **27**
Thalassemias, 196, **197**
Thermal burn, 58, **59**
Thrombocytopenic purpura, 198, **199**
Thyroglossal duct cyst, 98, **99**
Tongue, bifid, 6, **7**
– crenated, 84, **85**
– diseases, 80–87
– fissured, 82, **83**
– geographic, 80, **81**
– hairy, 82, **83**
Trauma, factitious, 40, **41**
– toothbrush, 40, **41**
Traumatic hematoma, 40, **40**
– neuroma, 272, **273**
– ulcer, 38, **38, 39**
Torus mandibularis, 8, **9**
– palatinus, 8, **9**
Toxic epidermal necrolysis, 170, **171**
Trichloroacetic acid burn, 50, **51**
Tuberculosis, 132, **133**

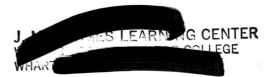

Tuberous sclerosis, 28, **28**, **29**
Tumor, acinic cell, 238, **239**
– granular cell, 274, **274**
– like lesions, 293–297
– melanotic neuroectodermal of infancy, 286, **287**
– mucoepidermoid, 240, **241**
Tumors, benign, 264–290
– metastatic, 250, **250**, **251**

U

Ulcer, eosinophilic, 48, **49**
– lingual frenum, after cunnilingus, 42, **43**
– traumatic, 38, **38, 39**
Ulceration due to azathioprine, 62, **63**
– due to methotrexate, 62, **63**
Ulcers, aphthous, major, 150, **151**
– – minor, 149, **149**
– – recurrent, 149
– herpetiform, 150, **151**

V

Varicella, 104, **105**
Varices, sublingual, 86, **87**

Vegetans, pemphigus, 174, **174**
Verruca vulgaris, 108, **109**
Verruciform xanthoma, 272, **273**
Verrucous carcinoma, 234, **235, 236**
– hyperplasia, 264, **265**
Vitiligo, 192, **193**

W

Warthy dyskeratoma, 192, **193**
Wegener's granulomatosis, 156, **157**

X

Xanthoma verruciform, 272, **273**
Xanthomas, 202, **203**
Xeroderma pigmentosum, 228, **229**
Xerostomia, 292, **292**

Z

Zoster, herpes, 102, **103**